Dead Medics' Society

by Mike Albany

tfm Publishing Ltd, Castle Hill Barns, Harley, Nr Shrewsbury, SY5 6LX, UK.
Tel: +44 (0)1952 510061; Fax: +44 (0)1952 510192
E-mail: nikki@tfmpublishing.com; Web site: www.tfmpublishing.com

Design and layout: Nikki Bramhill

Copyright © Mike Albany 2005
Illustrator Andy White
Front cover image courtesy of NASA: Hubble Space Telescope Center

ISBN 1 903378 34 6

Apart from any fair dealing for the purposes of research or private study, or criticism or review, as permitted under the Copyright, Designs and Patents Act 1988, this publication may not be reproduced, stored in a retrieval system or transmitted in any form or by any means, electronic, digital, mechanical, photocopying, recording or otherwise, without the prior written permission of the publisher.

Neither the authors, nor the publisher, nor any other party who has been involved in the preparation or publication of this work can accept responsibility for any injury or damage to persons or property occasioned through the implementation of any ideas or use of any product described herein. Neither can they accept any responsibility for errors, omissions or misrepresentations, howsoever caused.

Printed by Gutenberg Press Ltd., Gudja Road, Tarxien, PLA 19, Malta.
Tel: +356 21897037; Fax: +356 21800069.

Dedication

To Nikki, my editor at tfm, for trusting me.

To begin: a little anatomy

The single large artery carrying blood away from your heart is called the aorta - the main highway of the arterial system. Every minute, about the time it will take you to sit quietly and read this page, all the blood in your body - that's five litres, or eight pints - circulates back to the heart, passes through your lungs to pick up oxygen, and gets pumped out into the aorta again. At about an inch in diameter it is somewhat wider than a garden hose, and arches backwards within the chest before coming to lie next to the spine. Smaller branches coming off the aortic arch supply high pressure arterial blood to the right arm, the head and neck via the right and left carotid arteries (so beloved of macabre thriller writers), and finally, a branch to the left arm. Thereafter, the aorta runs down in front of the backbone and pierces the diaphragm to enter the abdomen, where further branches supply blood to the spleen, liver, guts, kidneys and pancreas, until at about the level of the belly button, it neatly forks into two; one branch to each leg.

As one might imagine, like a hosepipe used continuously night and day for fifty years or more, with age the aorta tends to weaken in places and expand. Weak expanded segments are called aneurysms, from the Greek *aneurusma*, meaning "dilatation". Interestingly, and to diverge for a moment, comparative anatomists have suggested the structure of the aorta in different animals - including man - correlates with the life expectancy of that particular species.

In other words, it seems the thickness and elasticity of the aortic wall has built-in redundancy; it is doomed to lose its integrity towards the end of a normal lifespan and become aneurysmal. Of course, like an old hosepipe expanding and thinning, an aneurysm can only balloon out so far, before it bursts...

1

Blood. Warm blood and guts. David Gray was up to his elbows in both, though experience told him things were cooler than they should be. He could feel it through his fingertips and the back of his hands. At two in the morning he'd already been at it an hour and the patient was getting cold; hardly surprising after such a massive transfusion.

'How much has he had?' he asked the gas man at the top end of the table.

'Ten units of blood, two litres of colloid, two of crystalloid, six fresh frozen plasmas - oh yeah, some platelets too. How are you doing?'

'Bottom end's nearly on. Give me ten minutes and the clamp'll be off.'

He'd been doing aneurysms for close on thirty years; thousands of them. Why did the leaking ones always come in at night? This one was seventy-two and fit; at least that's what the registrar told him over the phone, forcing him from bed for a double-quick drive to the hospital. 'Get him to theatre then,' he had sighed wearily, 'I'll be there in twenty minutes.'

By the time Gray had changed and scrubbed the patient was already on the table, and except for the abdomen, completely hidden beneath green drapes. The whole team was there; anaesthetists, junior surgeons to assist, scrub nurses, runners, technicians. Almost a dozen, and for what? A fifty-fifty chance the guy might survive.

That's the trouble with emergency triple As: abdominal aortic aneurysms. Planned operations are worthwhile because most survive. Burst ones drop dead on the spot, or at least ninety-five percent do; pumping your entire circulating blood volume into your belly tends to have that effect. A few hang on long enough to get to a hospital, but even then, despite surgery, half of them still die; either bleeding to death on the table, or suffering multi-organ failure after days or weeks of torture on a ventilator in the intensive care unit.

Right now, he had clamps on the aorta above and below the ruptured segment and was repairing it by implanting a Dacron tube graft, much as a plumber does with a split pipe, though Gray had to sew rather than solder the cloth-like prosthesis in place. Before completing the anastomosis with a few final sutures, he briefly released the clamps to "blow" the graft through; a hissing gush of pressurized arterial blood leaping scarlet into the air to dislodge any clots.

'Okay, Bill, I'm ready when you are.'

'Let me fill him up a bit first, Dave.' The anaesthetist turned all the IV lines on full, and holding both hands up high on the drip stands, squeezed the plastic bags hard, forcing in more fluid and blood. Once the clamps came off the blood pressure would fall as the legs and lower body came back into the circulation. It was always a tricky few minutes, balancing the fluid deficit and haemodynamics against the need for the heart to pump harder and faster. Get it wrong and there was a danger of stroke or heart attack as the blood pressure went too high or too low. 'Right, try it now,' he said after a minute.

Gray removed the clamps and fixed his gaze on the wall-mounted blood pressure monitor, the digital read-out linked directly to the patient's left wrist and radial artery. He stood in a self-assured relaxed poise, one bloodied hand resting on his hip, the other still within the open abdomen, fingers poised to compress the graft closed should the pressure drop.

Seventy; too low; pinch.

Ninety now and Bill was still pushing in blood. Gray's practised eyes observed everything; release again, let the legs fill up. Seventy; pinch. Five minutes later the patient was stable. Pressure one-twenty, no bleeding from the suture line.

'Any urine?'

A nurse checked the catheter bag. 'Nothing yet.'

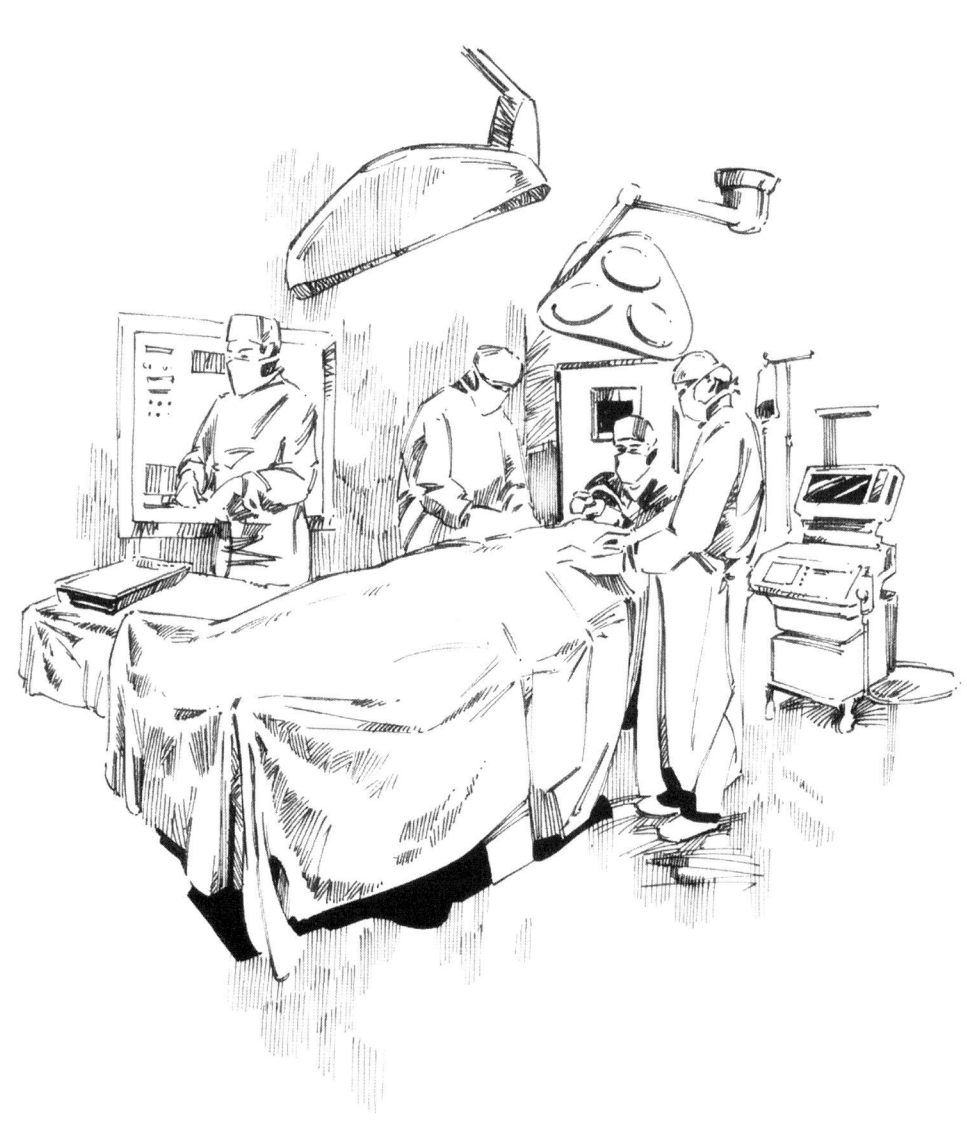

Damn it, he thought. Once through the operation, kidney failure was probably the biggest killer. If the guy didn't pee soon he wasn't going to; the start of a slippery slope.

'Close him up then,' he directed the registrar. 'And let's not take all night over it, eh! While you're doing that, I'll do the notes.'

Alone in the theatre rest room and still in greens, Gray wearily dropped the patient's file onto one of the coffee tables, slumped his lean body into a nearby armchair, threw back his head, and sighed in dismay. He imagined a daily trek to the ICU over the coming week, the bad news getting worse at every visit: "No urine yet, Mr Gray, the renal boys want to dialyse him"; "No chance of getting him off the ventilator, he's still on full inotrope support"; "Liver function's off the clock, might be time to call it a day." Pulling the blue theatre cap from his head, he ran both hands slowly through his hair before massaging his face. It was all so bloody frustrating and depressing.

He flicked idly through the admission notes: *Alfred Angel, 72, retired labourer, unmarried, lives alone, previously fit, no relatives, no dependants, non-smoker, non-drinker. Found collapsed by neighbour.* Ah well, at least there wouldn't be any anxious relatives to placate with comforting platitudes. But with no family in support, if the man survived he'd need a whole raft of social services to get him back home. And what then? A slow decline into a miserable, lonely old age?

Leaning back in the chair, hands clasped behind his neck, he blew air through pursed lips. What a waste of time! All the effort and expense. Whichever way it went, Alfred Angel was going to be a loser. 'Poor bastard would be better off dead,' he muttered to the ceiling. 'When it's my turn just give me Scotch and diamorph, then leave me be.'

Gray hung around until about three-thirty to see the patient safely transferred to an ICU bed, plugged into a ventilator and ensnared in a tangle of intravenous lines and monitor leads. Then he changed, thankfully found his car where he'd left it under the lights outside casualty - theft or break-ins weren't unknown in the shadows of the main car park - and headed back home. The junior staff all had rooms at the city hospital when they were on-call and could take care of things till morning. In any case, he had to get home if only to shower and get into a suit and tie; after the registrar's phone call, for speediness he'd chucked on some old jeans and a sweat-shirt, but with a full day's work still ahead, respectable attire was required.

There was still time for bed though. And the warm safe haven of his wife's arms, even if it was only for a couple of hours. Poor long-suffering Kate, her night's rest would be as equally disturbed as his own, yet she wouldn't complain - never had done in all the years they'd been married. Even way back in the early days, when he was a junior doctor and she was a part-time nurse, living cooped-up in grotty little hospital flats, with the kids, no money, and the phone constantly summoning him to work. Gray envisaged the forthcoming scene, repeated more times than he cared to recall: creeping into the darkened bedroom, quietly undressing, slipping in beside her as she feigned sleep, and then the warm softness against his bare chest when she scuttled across the sheets to lie next to his body with a whispered, "How did it go?" As always he'd gently scold her for staying awake until his return, and with a wicked grin she'd say it was her duty as his present wife and lover to wait up for the master of the house, otherwise he might be tempted to get a different model. Then she'd nuzzle into his neck with a kiss and promptly close her eyes.

Yes, back to bed - he smiled at the thought - though he doubted sleep would come. There was always the chance he'd get called out again for something else, or have to give advice over the phone. And middle-of-the-night aneurysms never failed to leave his nerves jangling like a steel band on speed. As a young man he could cat-nap on a washing line, yet be instantly awake and alert when necessary, but now at fifty-eight, his old bones took longer to settle and even longer to spring into action.

With one hand on the steering wheel Gray cracked the driver's window an inch, reached into a pocket and rewarded his night's efforts with a slim panatella, lighting it and blowing smoke in one quick adept action. Five a day he allowed himself; or rather Kate did. It used to be cigarettes, but she'd cajoled him into finally giving up when he hit his half-century. The cigars were a compromise for when he badly needed a nicotine hit, like now: "But promise me no more than five a day. And not in the house!" And he could never break a promise to Kate.

His reverie ranged unfettered - as it tended to do when driving alone in the middle of the night - and the latest member of the family sidled into his imaginings. They had a grandson at last, just three weeks ago, and he couldn't have wished for a better Christmas present. Young Toby; he liked the name, it had a good solid ring to it. Kate had wept tears of joy at the news, soaking the handpiece of the phone before handing it over to him, clap-dancing on the spot, and then immediately demanding it back again. All he'd managed was a hurried "Well done, love," before Kate was giving instructions and asking questions once more. His youngest daughter, his darling baby girl, and now she was the mother of his first grandson. Jeez, he was changing her nappies only yesterday, where had all those years gone? Still, no matter, now he could do all the things he'd wanted to do with the son they never had. Teach him to fish, definitely; take him to the rugby, the football, the cricket, and perhaps one day, even the pub! He laughed out loud to himself before sucking and blowing more aromatic smoke. They were coming over on Sunday for lunch, all three daughters with families in tow to celebrate Toby's arrival. Kate had arranged it, and he was looking forward to it. He'd curb his enthusiasm till then.

The triple A man's fate didn't worry him. In fact he rarely worried over any patient these days. There wasn't much he hadn't seen before, wasn't any illness or disease his experience couldn't sniff out, wasn't any operation in his field he couldn't do as well or better than the next man. And that was the trouble, he mused - boredom. It just wasn't exciting anymore. At sometime over all those years, surgery had become a production-line treadmill: hernias, gallbladders, colons, veins, stomachs, breasts, or anything else that came his way. When did it happen? God only knows. It just sneaked up on him, like that old man he saw shaving every morning in the bathroom mirror. Where in hell's name had *he* come from?

Chapter 1

The broad rower's shoulders were still there but slightly stooped - courtesy of countless hours leaning over operating tables - and the once firm muscles had turned flabby, with cropped salt and pepper hair, creases around the eyes, worry lines, receding hairline and gums - the whole caboodle.

Then there were the on-calls, like tonight. Thirty years ago it was every other night and his body could cope with it easily; now it was only once a week and every fifth weekend, but the constant stone-in-the-shoe feeling of waiting for the phone to ring always left him drained. And how much of his life had surgery stolen away? Too much for sure. All he wanted now was to make it through to the finish - strange to think of it as some sort of sentence - and retire.

Yet there was a time when becoming a "cutter" consumed his every thought, when the only goal of his life was to be a consultant surgeon like his old bosses. Those guys were astounding and inspirational. On ward rounds they'd stand at the foot of the bed and make a diagnosis just by looking into the patient's face. It was uncanny and fascinating. He smiled at the memory:

"Tell me the history again if you would, Doctor Gray"; "Mm, yes. And what did you find on examination?" A moment's thought, perhaps even - lo and behold - a hand on the patient's abdomen. "I don't care what all the tests say, this man has ...".

And whatever it was, they'd be right.

Now he could do it himself. It *was* there in the face, every time. Or in the eyes. Or in the voice of a concerned and worried junior who suddenly found himself out of his depth. You can't teach experience, or the sixth sense that comes with it.

Pity.

And could they operate! Geniuses with their hands. Or so it seemed at the time. Now he knew it was all down to experience again: how hard to pull, when to cut with gay abandon, when to dissect gently. When to rant and rave at the juniors or scrub nurses to get the best out of them - all an act of course. He did that as well. Not by way of imitation though. It just happened. Came with the territory. With the years.

Alone with his thoughts, Gray steered the Jaguar saloon along the familiar and deserted roads at a more leisurely pace than a few hours previously. The January air was crisp and clear, with no cloud cover and a sharp frost, but the gentle warm blower kept him snugly cocooned against the silky-black night.

The aneurysm man drifted back into his mind. Would he live or die? Stupid question: of course he would die, everyone dies in the end, don't they? Sure, but would he get over the operation: yes or no? And did he care? He pondered the question only briefly before whispering the answer into the darkness.

'He'll either make it or he won't. I've given it my best shot and he's had his chance, so it's up to him now. And his kidneys.'

Gray chuckled to himself at the amusing postscript and carefully negotiated a road junction. If everyone dies in the end, why then was he bothering?

'"To relieve pain and suffering my boy",' he mimicked the rich baritone of one of his old professors, then added, 'Pompous arse.'

Of course there was an element of truth in the statement, but how perverse is it to relieve pain and suffering with a knife? Okay, there's trauma; surgery can help if you've been run over by a bus. But aneurysms? No symptoms at all apart from the emotional anxiety of being told you've got one, and the pain, suffering, and risk to life and limb of having it fixed. And what about cancer? The layman's perception is it must be cut out early - before it spreads - whereas it's a fact most cancers have already metastasised far and wide by the time they're diagnosed.

Breast cancer was a particular hobby horse of Gray's. A hundred years ago surgeons would compete to do the widest excisions possible, even going so far as forequarter amputations - breast, arm and shoulder blade, complete with all the muscles and lymph nodes - in the mistaken belief that cancer spread in a logical radial progression outwards. In his youth Gray had seen the results of supra-radical mastectomy; little old ladies who survived long enough to teach him to curse his predecessors for performing such butchery. The mere fact the women were alive after so many years was an indication the original diagnosis was probably incorrect: they never had cancer in the first place.

Nowadays everyone knew cancerous breast cells disseminated throughout the body at the onset, and cutting out the primary did nothing to prevent the malign fatality of secondary spread. He wanted to shout back through the ages: 'It's already happened, stupid. The horse has bolted! The only hope is the body's immune system, or blunderbuss systemic chemotherapy to poison the cells in their hidey-holes.'

Was he mutilating patients himself? Had he? Undoubtedly yes, and in a hundred years his successors would brand him a butcher also, and want to yell back at him. How depressing! What then was the answer? He didn't know. He was resigned simply to do his best, though even that had changed.

As a young man and a young surgeon, Gray never doubted his actions. He was a trained professional who could challenge any surgical illness with a knife and arrogant, unswerving self-confidence. Like the archetypal surgeon's epitaph which so amused his physician colleagues:

> ***Here lies Sir Archibald Arbuthnot Slagg-Heepe FRCS***
> ***Seldom correct, but never in doubt***

Thankfully, his experience had brought with it a deep humility, deeper questions, and unlike the apocryphal Sir Archibald, unfathomable doubts. Gray never tired of reminding the juniors that every patient who ever had surgery by his hand would die: 'Remember this, even an in-growing toenail operation has a hundred percent mortality - eventually.'

He could tell by their bemused expressions they thought him a daft old sod whose time had passed. Perhaps he was and perhaps it had. But in their fresh young faces he recognised himself at the same age, full of knowledge and new-found skills with a burning urge to apply them without forethought or consideration: the patient has a lump and I have an operation, therefore, the two must come together. Now he was wise enough to look over and beyond the parapet. What was that saying? Wisdom is the jockey on the horse of knowledge. Yes, that was it exactly. He knew how to steady and rein in the steed, to hold back on the bit with a firm gentle touch, to gain balance and control before finally, and irrevocably, leaping over the fence.

And who had taught him such fine horsemanship over all those long years? Why, his patients of course! The disappointment of seeing them come back with liver secondaries five years after "curative" bowel surgery. Recognising a patient on the stroke ward being spoon fed: "You did his aneurysm a couple of years ago, Mr Gray." The thankyou card to say Uncle Harry died from heart failure, but at least the Big C didn't come back to get him. One way or another they all succumbed, inevitably and inescapably, to their own mortality. And there was nothing he or surgery could do about it. He tried to put it all out of his mind, but the rock in his chest felt heavier than usual.

ooooooooooooooooooooooooooooooooo

The fox lifted its nose and sniffed the still night air once more. He was fit, handsome, and healthy. It was his second winter, and so far, migrating to the urban sprawl from the surrounding cold and barren countryside had been a great success. He'd found nirvana and thrived: a warm safe nest beneath a garden shed to sleep during the day and endless restaurants competing for his custom every evening, each one waiting for him there at the end of his snout. All he needed to do was follow the most alluring scent, and yes, there it was again; chicken bones.

It was unfortunate, as many happenstances are, that as Gray was evaluating his role in the great mysteries of life, death and surgery, the unwitting fox, enjoying the freedom darkness brings such creatures, chose such a moment to follow its nose and cross the Queen's highway. It was doubly unfortunate that one of its regular nocturnal foraging points included the dustbins of residences built on a malicious blind bend, with the added drawback of there being a dip in the road's surface which had a tendency to gather moisture.

Gray slammed on the brakes and turned the wheel; a reflex response without thought or consideration, and born out of kindliness to all of Mother

Nature's creations. And yet, in the final analysis, it was inherently stupid because brakes and rubber need a good surface on which to purchase and accomplish their task.

The frosty night, the dew point, the ice, the canine eyes glowing silver-red in the headlamp beams, the low coefficient of friction, the timeline joining them all, karma, chance, lack of sleep, fate, serendipity...

Whatever.

In short, the Jaguar's offside front wheel hit the kerbstone first, flinging the vehicle into space, and the rear wheel hit a millisecond later, imparting a rotational moment. Thus it was that after take-off the car adopted a gentle parabolic trajectory, spinning all the while around its longitudinal axis.

In all, not dissimilar to a shell - a metallic finish midnight-blue shell with chrome trim - rifling from a field gun.

14 Dead Medics' Society

2

Still in his jeans and sweat-shirt, Gray stood at the front of the small crowd gathered on the sidewalk. The others were variously dressed in nightgowns, coats, or whatever else they managed to grab while hastily exiting their beds to survey the scene. Across the road beyond the police cordon, fire, ambulance and rescue crews laboured amongst the wreckage.

The front wall and corner of the house was partly collapsed onto the crushed and upturned Jaguar. Cracks in the remaining brickwork, illuminated by the harsh halogen arc-lamps set up in the small garden, spread upwards to the first floor and around the sagging bedroom windows. The whole façade was perilously dangerous and unstable, yet men were feverishly shifting rubble and glass from the car even as steel props were being jacked into place. Police road blocks a hundred yards to either side of the crash site intermittently bathed the unfolding drama with blue and red tints of flashing colour.

A woman to one side of Gray, a duvet slung around her shoulders against the bitter cold, silently moved her lips in prayer.

'Is anybody in there?' Gray asked her, concerned his skills might be of use to any residents trapped within the house. But she didn't reply. Her eyes remained fixed on the carnage, praying still.

It was his car, no question about it; he recognised the number plate, inverted and poking out from where the front door of the house should be. But - he looked himself over, feeling for bruises or broken bones - there wasn't a mark on him. Must have been thrown clear then, he reconciled. No pain, not even a scratch. No dirt either, his soft hands still looked freshly scrubbed, nails perfectly manicured. How was that?

An elderly man in pyjamas appeared from the rear of the assembly and spoke directly to Gray, 'Shame about yer motor.' There was a sad tone to his rough voice and manner, as if genuinely upset. 'Lovely it was, really smooth ride. Luxury leather seats, cruise control, all mod cons. Completely buggered now though ain't it? Scrap value only, I reckon. Still, no harm done and you'll be well insured. Right?'

'Yes,' Gray replied, incredulous that anyone would want to pass such comment. 'But what about the house!' He nodded towards the bomb-site opposite. Paramedic crews were still risking their necks underneath tottering masonry. 'Is it yours?'

'Oh no, mate, not mine. The couple who live there are away. Spain I think. Winter sun, that sorta thing,' he said, scratching at his silvery chin stubble.

'Thank God for that.' Gray breathed a sigh of relief. 'No-one's hurt then.'

'Nah, not really. Spectacular crash though wasn't it?'

'I don't remember much of it. There was a fox, I think, and skidding... Hold on a minute, all those men over there, do they know the house is empty?'

'Course they do.'

'Well why in hell's name are they risking themselves like that? I've got to tell them I'm here. That I'm safe!'

Gray set off towards the house but the man in pyjamas, his feet bare, jumped forward and held him by the shoulder. 'Best not get in their way, David. You don't mind me calling you by your first name do you? Let them get on with their job.'

'They haven't got a job have they?' Gray shouted and pointed to his car. 'I'm not over there, am I?' He slapped his chest, 'I'm here!'

By now they were standing in the middle of the road, and as he remonstrated, from the crash site a traffic cop in an orange Dayglo vest and hard hat trotted towards them both. Gray turned to face him, expecting a rebuke for approaching too close. 'Officer,' he said, holding his arms outstretched like a supplicant, 'it's my car, there's no need to risk...'

But the cop ran straight past and started urging the crowd back to their beds. Gray addressed the pyjama man again. 'Did you see that? The bloody fool

Chapter 2

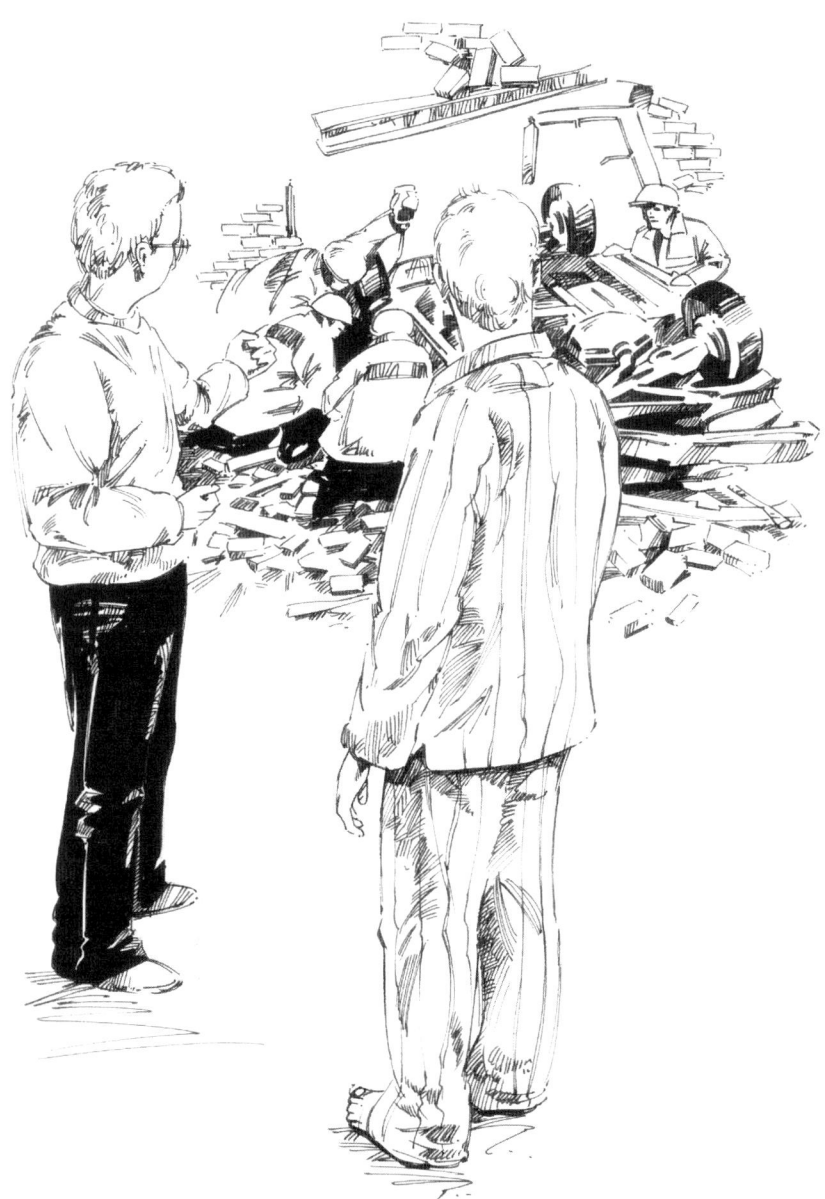

ignored me,' and before waiting for an answer, marched off to tackle the recalcitrant lawman. 'Officer, officer! Listen to me man, are you deaf or something?'

But there was no answer. The faces in the crowd, a mixture of anxiety and bloodthirsty curiosity, took no notice of him either. Law-abiding citizens all, they grumbled quietly and started shuffling back to their homes. Gray gently tapped the rear of the Dayglo vest with a fingertip. Still no response. 'Officer!' he bellowed, urgently grabbing at the policeman's upper arm, intending to physically jerk him around.

But there was no resistance. As if trying to grasp at a hologram, Gray's hand clutched seemingly at thin air. Momentarily stunned, he examined his palm, blinked a few times, and tried again. And again. Nothing! He could see the man, see the uniform, discern the shape of a policeman, but there was nothing to feel. Then the obvious solution came to him. It was all a dream.

It must be. Had to be.

"Fraid not, me old son,' the pyjama man said calmly from behind him.

Generally a man of cool nerve and calculated actions, Gray jumped and spun around like a startled rabbit. 'You still here?' he said, for want of something better to say in a dream.

The man shrugged his shoulders and stuck out his lower lip in an exaggerated "Why not?" sort of pose. But Gray wasn't having any of it. He was in control again, though in an exceptionally surreal way.

'Look chum, this has to be a dream. This young copper here can't see or feel me because he isn't real. He's not even solid. Watch this!' Gray stroked his hand through the officer's midriff before bringing his index finger to bear at eye level, jabbing it with emphasis. 'And you! You're standing there in tatty old pyjamas and bare feet on a night like this. I reckon you'd better get yourself back indoors before you catch your death. Meanwhile, I'm going to take a stroll until I wake up.' He turned and began walking in the direction of home.

'David Gray. Wait! We need to talk.'

Chapter 2

There was an insistence in the shouted command that Gray found compelling, even overwhelming. He stopped and turned back.

The man was fingering the threadbare and faded material of the jacket. 'It's not my fault they're tatty, the hospital put them on me.'

'What did you say?'

'I said the hospit…'

'Yes, yes, I heard what you said. What I mean is, what are you talking about, and how do you know my name?'

'David,' he sighed. 'Or do you like, Dave, better?'

'Whatever.' Gray furtively pinched the skin at the top of his thigh. He could feel it. It hurt. This was like no dream he'd ever experienced.

'You look more of a Dave to me. My name's Alf, by the way. We haven't been properly introduced.' He held out his hand.

From ingrained politeness Gray reciprocated, and the two shook. 'Pleased to meet you,' he muttered, though in truth, he didn't care less. Any minute now he was going to wake up in bed and this nightmare would be over. Are you supposed to feel pain in a dream, or not? He tried to remember.

Alf had a big hand, a big workman's hand, and held his firm grip longer than was socially necessary. Then he squeezed, hard enough to make Gray wince. 'Can you feel that, Dave? Is it uncomfortable? Am I solid enough for you?'

'Yeeeeow. Stop. Please stop it. Now.'

'Huh!' Alf guffawed and let go, palm up. 'Still think yer dreamin' now?'

Alarmed - more at the implications of the discomfort in his hand rather than the sensation - and wanting to distance himself from any further physical contact with this strange madman called Alf, the surgeon stepped two paces backwards, and instantly vanished into the policeman, where his world turned abruptly and opaquely red. Fearful and disorientated, he also felt irritation, but sensed it wasn't his own. Gray's temporary host wanted the shift finished, the rubber-neckers to clear the pavement, the stiff in the car extricated so they could clear up the mess and bring in the demolition team, to win the lottery, to screw the new typist back at the station, a promotion, a fried breakfast, a smoke, a beer... Gray leapt forward, literally shocked out of the policeman's skin. Jesus! What was happening?

Alf was waiting for him to reappear, bent over double, hands on knees, laughing so much there were tears in his eyes. 'Dave,' he gasped, 'that's got to be the funniest thing I've seen in years, your face is a bloody picture. Yer arms were stickin' out of 'is shoulder blades like 'is 'ead was on backwards. Yer should 'ave seen it.'

Gray scrutinised the man's features carefully, but saw only honesty. 'This *is* real, isn't it?' His tone sounded overly controlled, an attempt to subdue the panic fermenting in his chest. He knew he was in trouble. In need of help. And Alf, this lunatic with uncommonly blue eyes and tears of mirth rolling down his wrinkled cheeks, seemed the only option available.

By the time Alf stopped slapping his thighs and pleading with Gray to do the vanishing trick again, the crowd had more or less dispersed, and the unsavoury policeman was back with his chums at the crash site.

'Yes, Dave, it's real,' Alf said, verging on laughter once more.

'But it can't be! What's going on?'

Alf sucked on his teeth, suddenly serious, and eyed Gray up and down as if contemplating something of great portent. 'Follow me,' he said finally. 'But please, Dave, please try an' stay calm.'

The old man - for that is how Gray perceived his new acquaintance, forgetting that no man ages between the ears - walked briskly across the road towards the house opposite, hesitating momentarily in front of the barricade before apparently deciding to walk around it. Once in the garden, beyond the open gate, the pair stood among the rescue workers on the lawn, totally unchallenged and totally unseen.

'They don't know we're here!' Gray whispered.

'No,' Alf said vaguely, his concentration elsewhere. He crouched down on his haunches, peering through and around the debris, searching for something. 'There you are. Look,' he said with satisfaction, pointing a finger through the

Chapter 2

gaggle of paramedics surrounding the fusion of twisted metal and brickwork. Gray bent down to squint in the direction indicated, and his heart skipped several beats.

That's if he had a heart of course, but who can know for sure? It certainly felt like it to him. His mouth went dry as well, though that particular sensation can be a cheap hypnotist's deception foisted on the mind - no mouth necessary. Anyway, Gray's heart skipped several beats and his mind, or his consciousness, told him his mouth was dry.

He spied his own body, bloodied and bent and upside down in the driver's seat, an oxygen mask on his face and an IV line in his neck, the only part of his anatomy the paramedics could access.

It was expected. You expected it. Gray, though stunned at the prospect, suspected it. And naturally, we all thought Alf was better informed.

'I'm dead then,' Gray said with a cold finality.

'I honestly don't know, Dave.' Alf stood up, his knees cracking loudly with what sounded like arthritis.

'Well that's me there, yet I'm here. And I look as if I'm dead over there. What other answer is there?'

'You can't be dead yet, Dave, otherwise they wouldn't still be working on you would they? After all, you're the doc, you'd know better than me.'

Confused to the point of putting his fingertips up to where he felt his temples should be, Gray challenged the man. 'Who the hell are you, Alf? I thought you knew what was happening here?'

'Ain't yer got it yet?'

'Got what?'

'You were operatin' on me a few hours ago.'

'I beg your pardon?'

'Honest! I saw it all. Buggered if I know how, but there I was standing next to you. Just found myself there, watching everything. All that blood in my body. Amazing!' He shook his head in disbelief. 'Hey, you're damned good ain't you, a real expert! Oh yeah, that reminds me, what gives you the right to think I'd be better off dead?'

'You! That was you I... You heard me?'

'Dave, don't get so embarrassed me old mate. I agree with you. You did a fine job, but you're right, I would be better off dead. Fact is my life has been a bit, how do you say it, tedious, yeah that's the word, a bit tedious of late. No job see, nowt to get out of bed for and nothing to keep me there. No little woman to warm me, no family to look after. This is great though, ain't it? Don't feel the cold like I used to, don't feel hungry either. And I don't feel lonely no more, not with this lot following me around.' Alf jerked a thumb over his shoulder.

Although the crowd of on-lookers had largely dispersed, beyond the police cordon there remained a small group dressed in rather old-fashioned workaday clothes, standing around and talking quietly among themselves. One of them, a prissy fiftyish looking woman with silver-grey hair tied up in a bun, a full-length black skirt and white neck-high blouse, left the others and strode fussily across the road, through the barriers, through the garden wall, and halted in front of Gray. His mouth fell open, slack-jawed in astonishment.

'Ignore my son,' the woman said bluntly. 'He's an idiot I'm afraid. Loveable, but an idiot just the same. Always has been and always will be. You are not dead, Mr Gray, and neither are you dreaming. This is real, or at least one aspect of reality, and these good people,' she indicated the surrounding firecrew and paramedics, 'are working hard and risking their own lives to save you. For a short time your spirit has been allowed freedom from any physical constraints. It is perhaps unfortunate that your companion and guide will be Alfred here, but you chose him by your thoughts and actions this night, so it cannot be undone. However, in his defence I am allowed to tell you that he is, although he doesn't know it and certainly doesn't act the part, a wise old soul who's never done any harm. And that, Mr Gray, is the very least we should expect of anyone. Though I'm afraid many can't manage even that small concession.'

Chapter 2

Alf was aggrieved at the feisty intrusion, though the gravitas of his objection was diluted by the worn pyjamas and bare feet. 'Ma, I don't need your help thank you all the same. I love you dearly but I'm perfectly capable...'

'Alfred Angel!' she scolded, her tone matriarchal and overbearing, but with barely concealed affection. 'You are capable of many things, but you are certainly not yet perfect. Perfection is something to which many aspire, but few attain.'

'Yeah but ma.'

'No buts, Alfred, we may have eternity but it's time for you to get started.' As she spoke, her hitherto solid form began to fade, slowly and inexorably, until she was gone.

Gray stole a glance across the road; the others had disappeared as well.

'Family!' Alf tut-tutted, shaking his head. 'What would you do with 'em, eh? Anyway, I suppose the old girl's right. Tell me, Dave, what day is it?'

But Gray, unhearing, peered into empty space, trying to grasp the enormity, the sheer outrageous absurdity of what was happening to him.

'Dave, mate. Hey, I'm talking to you. What day is it?'

'Eh? Er, Tuesday. No! No sorry, it's Wednesday morning.' He looked at his left wrist, but the Rolex was missing.

Alf recognised the movement and tilted his head towards the wreckage. "Fraid that'll still be in your car with you. You get yer clothes but a watch is no use. Anyway, we'd best get on with it, eh?'

'With what?'

"Aven't a clue, Dave. They told me to stick to you like glue till I die.'

'You aren't dead either then?'

'Nah, not yet. I'm due for a heart attack on Friday. At least that's what they told me before the crash. We were all there you see, in the car, followin' you around after my operation.'

'Who were all there, and where?'

'My family. They came to collect me. Seems that's what 'appens. But they wanted me to do something first, before, y'know.'

'You called her an old girl just now. But your mother looks younger than you.'

'Suppose she is, but then I was only about ten when she died, so she'll always be "the old girl" you see, because that's what pa called her. Still does matter o' fact, and he died when he was eighty. Mind you, she's still the boss. None of us'll dare cross her. You've seen what she's like, tongue like a razor.'

Just then, somewhere deep between his ears, Gray heard her voice again. *"I am waiting gentlemen. Please do get on."*

3

Gray recognised the place immediately, though he had no clue as to how they got there, or why. It had been part of his domain a few months after qualifying, during his first job as a medical houseman. Was this some sort of memory trick?

A primitive coronary care unit from thirty years ago with six beds of the old-fashioned kind; cream-coloured heavy tubular constructions with a web of springs supporting each mattress. And because it was the heart ward, interposed between the mattress and springs of every bed was a wooden board the size of a door, its brown edge showing beneath each neatly tucked-in bedcover: a firm base for whenever external cardiac massage was required.

It was late evening because the lights were dimmed, though somehow Gray already knew it. Five patients were asleep, or pretending to be, in their respective beds, ECG scopes glowing green on the wall above each one, tracing regular and irregular rhythms. The last bed, the one in the corner nearest the door, was curtained off around a bright overhead lamp, and distorted shadows danced behind the light-blue material. The shadows were whispering.

'Where are we Dave?' Alf said in his normal loud voice, gazing intently around.

'Ssh. Keep it down, they'll hear us!'

'Course they won't.' Alf laughed. 'Look.' He clapped his hands together like a rifle shot, but there was no response. The gentle snoring and whispering continued as before.

Gray shook his head in exasperation. 'Well at least show some respect. These people are ill. Follow me.' He led the way to the curtained off bed, searching for a chink in the drapes to peek through into the cubicle. There wasn't one.

'Allow me.' Alf moved alongside Gray and bent forward from the waist. His head disappeared from the shoulders up, as if decapitated by the falling fabric.

Gray, wary of the nebulous nature of supposedly solid objects, closed his eyes - he didn't know why, it just seemed natural - and followed suit. Inside he opened them again and turned his head to find Alf's grinning face.

'Easy innit?'

The patient - a woman of around sixty, propped up on pillows with her head thrown back, mouth wide open and gasping in short bubbling breaths - was drowning in her own fluid-sodden lungs. A plastic oxygen mask dangled from her neck where she had dragged it from her face in a fruitless attempt to suck in more air. Her lips and tongue were disticly blue, and the pale skin of her forehead and upper chest glistened with beads of cold sweat.

Two doctors in white coats, their backs turned, huddled over the medical notes in one corner. At the bedside a bosomly Caribbean nurse lifted the oxygen mask and attempted to hold it over the woman's mouth and nose, but the terrified creature thrashed out like an animal, as if trying to swim to the surface from the depths of the watery tomb engulfing her.

'I've given her diuretics and morphine, Anthony, but the pulmonary oedema's getting worse. I don't know what else to do!'

One of the doctors was young and scruffy looking, with collar-length black hair, a tie at half mast, and fear in his eyes. The pockets of his creased white coat bulged with notepads, pens, torches, a bleep, stethoscope, reflex hammer, a drug formulary, an ECG crib book, and all the other clutter novice doctors hope will make up for inexperience. Gray recognised himself.

'Blimey Dave, you've still got bum fluff on yer chin,' Alf noted. 'What's goin' on?'

'I'm about to get an important lesson, so shut up and listen.'

The other doctor was older, thirty at least. Tall, manicured to perfection and suavely confident, Gray remembered him well: 'My name is Anthony, not Tony.' A senior registrar with ten years under his belt, not far off a consultant job, openly bored with the rigours of on-call duty, and nothing but a gold fountain pen spoiling the contours of his virginal white coat. He peered impassively at the patient and then at Gray, taking a quick glance at the namebadge on his lapel. 'Er, David, let's go into the corridor and have a chat.'

The young Gray, the old Gray and Alf, gathered in a semi-circle outside the ward, just beyond the swing doors with glass portholes, and all three hung on every word of Anthony's considered opinion.

'She's dying, David. Apart from giving her a new heart, there's nothing more you or anyone else can do. This is her fifth infarct and she hasn't any myocardium left to pump. Set up a morphine drip and sedate her, give her more frusemide if you like, but the main thing is to stop her suffering. Pulmonary oedema isn't a nice way to go.'

'But we *can't* let her die, Anthony,' the young Gray pleaded. This was *his* patient. He knew how to make her better. The books *told* him what to do, didn't they? He'd been talking to the woman earlier in the day when he admitted her. They'd been having a conversation for Christ's sake. 'We've got to do something!'

Anthony sighed deeply. 'This is your first one, isn't it?'

The young houseman looked to the floor and nodded dismally.

'Come on then, I'll give you a hand.'

Anthony led the way back into the dim ward. The doors swung open twice, but nobody noticed.

'He's a callous bastard, ain't he?' Alf said.

'Who says you have to care?' Gray mumbled as he followed in line. 'He was right, and good at his job.'

'You care! He doesn't.'

'Yes, but I'd only just started, hadn't I?'

'That sounds like an excuse to me. Nothing wrong in caring, is there?'

'Better to do a good job,' Gray snapped.

Back again around the woman's bed, it was clear she had deteriorated further during the minutes they were away. The struggling was over. Limp rather than calm, her eyes were closed and her breathing little more than desultory movements of the chest wall. With the inexorable lack of oxygen, she was succumbing to the inevitable, and asphyxiating.

'She's a-goin', doctors,' whispered the nurse in a sing-song Jamaican accent.

The ECG monitor showed the heart rate slowing.

'Looks like she's beaten us to it,' Anthony said quietly, aware the other patients in the ward would be straining to hear everything: the enclosed illusion of privacy behind the curtains was just that, an illusion. 'Feel for a pulse, David. While we're here you may as well pronounce her dead. Three minutes with no pulse or resps.'

The young houseman took her cold wrist and shook his head slowly. Then his fingers went to her clammy damp neck, feeling for the carotid. Nothing. It showed on his face, but there was puzzlement in his expression as well - the ECG trace was continuing to show its flicking rhythmic pattern. He looked to Anthony and then back at the monitor, indicating an unspoken question.

'Electrical complexes only, it doesn't mean the heart's pumping. It'll go on like that for some time, unless she starts...' as Anthony spoke the green line went crazy, zig-zagging across the screen, 'fibrillating. Like that.' He reached up and turned off the machine before continuing. 'Got an ophthalmoscope with you?'

Young Gray rummaged in his deep pockets, finally producing the instrument.

'What's that for, Dave?' Alf asked.

Old Gray, so transfixed by the well-remembered scene of his youth he could scarcely turn his head away, snatched a fleeting glance towards his inquisitive travelling companion, 'It's for looking in the eye,' and what he saw took his breath away. Or rather, would have done if he had lungs. But like his heart, who knows?

Chapter 3 **29**

Space within the curtained cubicle was at a premium. The nurse and two young doctors were on one side of the bed, Alf and Gray, invisible observers both, on the other. But now there were two others vying for standing room between him and Alf; a woman in a nightgown bearing an uncanny resemblance to the patient who was dying, and behind her, his hands on her shoulders, a balding man in his sixties wearing a three-piece suit. Both appeared in rude health. Gray flinched involuntarily.

The woman spoke first. 'I'm sorry to have startled you, but I just needed to say thanks before I go. You were so very kind, even though I could tell you were worried and frightened for me. Anyway here I am, so there's no need to fuss anymore. I'm in no pain and I'm back with my lovely husband.' She smiled up at him and patted one of his hands.

'That goes for me as well, doctor, you did a good job, so don't blame yourself,' her husband said. 'Come on now Mavis, we're not supposed to delay things like this. It's time to leave and I've lots to show you.'

The couple were still talking as they gradually became transparent and finally faded away. Gray reached out to where they had been, but his hand merely vanished through the curtain. He drew it back and peered at it, turned it over, touched his fingertips together a few times; they all seemed solid enough. Then an idea came to him, and he felt for his own pulse. There wasn't one. He half expected it.

'Alf,' he said, pointing to the woman on the bed. 'That was her, wasn't it?'

'You're catching on fast.'

'And her husband?'

'Yeah, he died some years back. He's been standing waiting with us for the last few minutes. Didn't you see her get up off the bed just now?'

Gray shook his head.

'Too interested in those two I suppose.' Alf nodded at the white coats.

Across the bed, the tutorial wasn't yet finished. 'Use the 'scope,' Anthony directed. 'Pupils should be fixed, dilated and unreactive to light.'

The young Gray lifted each eyelid in turn and shone the beam. Both eyes were as glassy and lifeless as a dead fish; the spark of her being was gone.

'Now look at the retina. If you're lucky, we're early enough to see tramlining in the central artery. Bubbles of nitrogen coming out of solution and floating in lines to the edge of the optic disc.'

There would be.

Old Gray remembered them - tiny silver bubbles moving along the artery like trains on a track - and recalled the emotions his young counterpart felt at that very moment, bent over the woman with his face an inch from her nose, trying to focus on the back of her eye. He had been angry and confused. Angry with the oh-so-cool senior registrar, a man so stuck up himself he insisted on "Anthony" rather than "Tony" like any normal bloke, and who showed no sympathy or remorse for a woman who a few minutes earlier had been a living breathing human being. For Anthony she had turned into a teaching aid. Most of all though, he had been angry at his own impotence, and confused by the futility of all the medicine he'd learned.

Yes, it was an important lesson. And the first and last time Gray ever looked for tramlining.

oooooooooooooooooooooooooooooooooo

It was another ward in the same hospital, a ward from the mid-seventies, the open Nightingale type with high ceilings and a row of beds along the length of both walls. Tall sash windows betrayed the late-Victorian ancestry of the architecture, and slanting shafts of dazzling sunlight illuminated the long hall-like room, picking out motes of dust dancing like powdered gold in the lazy air currents. Nurses in starched hats and crisp white aprons patrolled the patients - all women - under the watchful eagle-eye of sister, who was sitting imperiously at her desk near the entrance; though even she failed to spot Alf and Gray.

'What's going on, Alf? I recognise this place as well, it's the female medical ward. How did we get here?'

'Dunno mate. I've only been doing this a few hours longer than you, ain't I?' He shrugged his shoulders and looked around. 'I think we're supposed to be here though, otherwise I reckon we'd be somewhere else.'

'What the hell does "supposed to be here" mean? What's all this in aid of?'

'Keep yer shirt on, Dave. Like I told you, I dunno, do I! All the old girl said was for me to look after you, and that's what I'm doin'.'

'So you're not responsible for moving us around?'

'Nah, course not. I wouldn't know how, would I?'

'She said something about me choosing you by my thoughts and actions.'

'Ma talks funny that way, old fashioned like. Half the time she's way over my head.'

Gray studied his escort's open honest face, and concluded Alf was only slightly less confused than himself. He knew and appeared to trust his mother though, and she seemed to be the key to whatever was going on: "*My thoughts and actions*," he pondered, but could make no sense of it.

'Dave!' Alf interrupted Gray's daydreaming, and indicated the swing doors. 'Isn't that you again?'

A little less disheveled than previously and with more confidence in his step, young Gray strode onto the ward, spoke briefly with sister at her desk, and hurried into a side-room. Alf made to follow, but his companion was reluctant.

'What's up, Dave?'

'I'm not sure I want to see this, if it's what I think it is.'

But his wish went unheeded, for as before, in the blink of an eye, Gray and Alf were in the side-room observing the young doctor at work. The narrow bed held a slim Asian girl of no more than fifteen or sixteen. With long hair shining black as gunmetal against the white pillow, flawless olive skin, a fine jawline and high cheekbones, she was as beautiful and delicate as a butterfly's wing. But her eyes were closed; she was unconscious and unresponsive.

'Come on, Chitra, wake up. Please don't do this to me. Please!' The young Gray flung off the bedcovers and examined the girl frantically, his movements quick and skilful through months of practice; tapping reflexes with a rubber hammer, examining pupils, feeling muscle tone, stroking the soles of her bare feet with his thumbnail. The left big toe flicked upwards, the right went down.

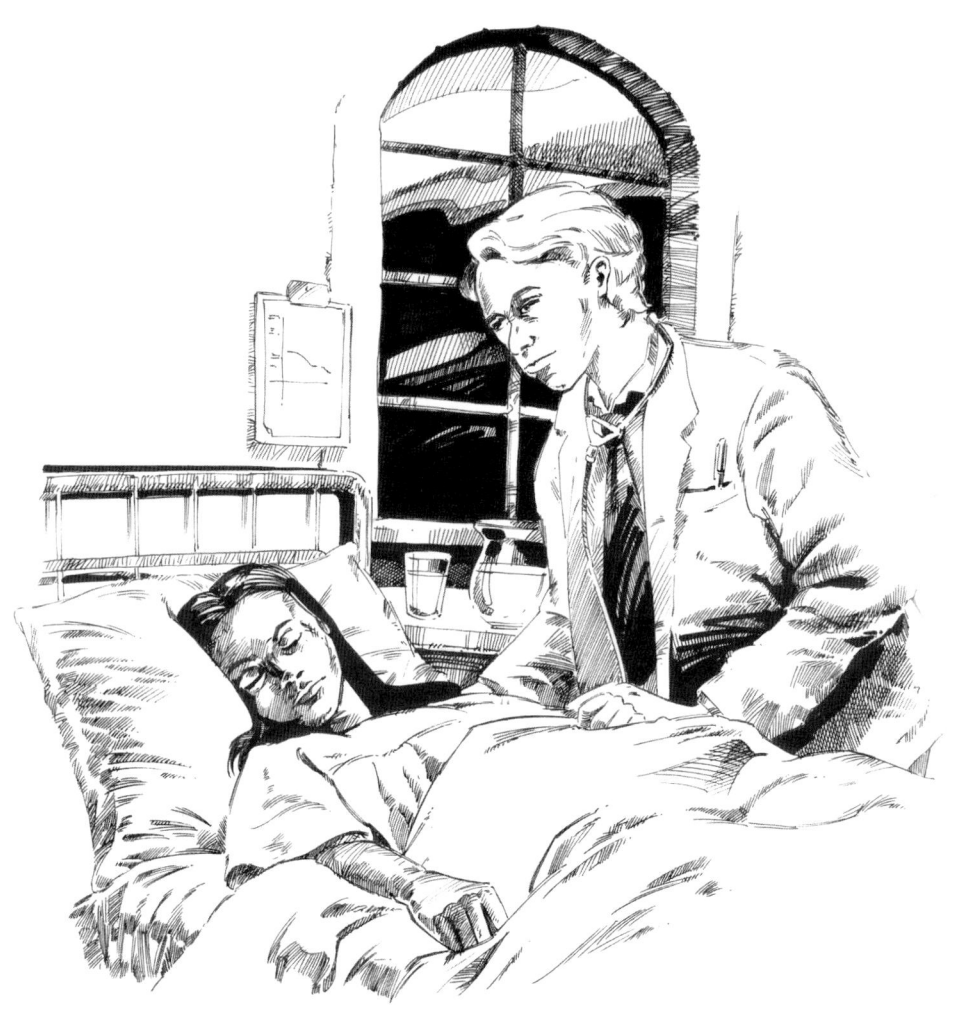

Chapter 3

'Shit, shit, shit,' he hissed to himself. Then seemingly in desperation, he knelt by the bed, stroked her head and spoke softly into her ear. 'Chitra, I know you're in there. Don't give up on me now. Fight it. I'm going to get some help, so don't you dare leave me. I'll be back soon.'

Alf watched the young man run out of the room, but old Gray's brimming eyes never left the girl.

'You okay, mate?' Alf ventured.

'No, Alf..., I'm not,' he sobbed. 'She never regained consciousness. That morning I was planning to send her home, and she...'

Gray hid his face in his hands as the sorrow bubbled like scum to the surface of his memory, and his shoulders shuddered for a few moments before the experienced veteran in him took control. When he opened his eyes again he was standing by a park bench in warm sunlight, with Alf hovering anxiously nearby.

'I'm sorry, Dave. Didn't think you still had it in you to get so upset. Let's have a break and talk about it.' He indicated the vacant wooden bench.

Gingerly and delicately, Alf sat on the bench as though his arthritis was playing up, whereas he was actually conducting an experiment. Unsure if his backside would feel any resistance or just float through the slats, he let himself down slowly and gently. When it held him he leant back and relaxed, face beaming with satisfaction. 'I think I'm getting the hang of this.'

Gray, still standing, checked out the park - children playing, people lazing on the grass, trees, flowerbeds, tennis courts, a bandstand - but didn't recognise anything. Then he sat down next to Alf, noting their presence was unseen and unheeded by passers-by, despite the fact his new friend was still in pyjamas. 'You understand what's happening?' he said, encouraged by Alf's statement.

'I reckon,' Alf expounded, eyes closed and face to the sun, 'it's all down to intentions. Yer can decide if something's solid or not, depending on what yer want to do with it.'

'What are you babbling on about, Alf. I thought you said you're getting the hang of it?'

'This bench old son! We're sitting on it, but we can walk through doors and walls and curtains. How's that, eh?' Alf looked across at Gray. 'Got to be intentions, ain't it? Logic see.' He tapped his temple with a finger.

Gray hadn't considered the implausibility of not being able to sit down, but Alf's deduction made him suddenly doubtful, and with the uncertainty came a slow but definite sinking feeling. He jumped to his feet with a start.

Alf considered voicing his thoughts regarding the "solid" ground on which his companion now stood, but decided it would be better to keep quiet. Instead, he stood up with a sigh. 'C'mon then, Dave, let's walk instead. Tell me about that girl just now. What was wrong with her?'

The pair strolled around the park as Gray recounted the tale. 'She was a Ugandan Asian, youngest daughter of a big family that Idi Amin kicked out. She'd been in for weeks, months, with bacterial endocarditis.'

'Slow down, Dave!'

'Sorry. An infection in her heart, germs on the heart valves and chambers with septicaemia. Bloody sick, intravenous antibiotics, hundreds of blood tests, needles, painful injections, horrible drugs, and through it all she never complained, not once. She was just a kid, Alf. A perfect fragile lovely child with huge brown eyes and a smile like sunshine, no matter what torture we put her through. The family used to bring food in for her, home-made curries in those round stainless-steel pots they use, and she always saved some for me. That was my ward you see, and every morning she'd be the first patient I'd check on. My favourite, if you like. Then one day I came in and she was like you saw her. Stroked out during the night. The nurses couldn't wake her up. Turned out she'd had a mycotic embolus to her brain.'

Alf lifted a censorial eyebrow.

'A vegetation, a lump of crap growing in her heart or on one of the valves flew off and lodged in her brain. Blocked off the blood supply. We put her in the intensive care unit on a ventilator but she was brain-dead. My boss turned her off a few days later. I went for a walk on my own like this and cried my eyes out. It broke my heart, Alf. She was so young and so brave.'

'You never got over it did you?' Alf observed sagely as Gray wiped his cheeks dry.

'No, I suppose not. But I haven't thought about her in years. Forgot all about her.'

'I reckon yer never really forget anything,' Alf intoned. 'I reckon you just bury it like a dog with a bone, then a whiff of something comes along and brings it all back. Ever noticed how certain smells do that? Stir up yer emotions like, bring back the feelings, the memories? Burnt toast does it for me every time. Has done all me life. It's me father's fault, he never could get it right, always burning it he was. Six kids clamouring for food with ma on 'er death bed and him struggling to keep us all going with burnt toast and dripping. Mind you, I didn't know it at the time.'

'Didn't know what?'

'That she were dyin', and he was struggling. I've understood it since though, thinking it over each time one of them went.'

'Who?'

'My pa, and brothers and sisters. I was the youngest. Hardly remember me ma, but we were a close family. I was always treated like the kid until one by one they all died and left me on my own. Least I was on me own, until I got sick and you operated on me. Then they all appeared again. Look behind you.'

Gray glanced over his shoulder while keeping pace with Alf. Twenty yards behind, the path was filled with the same people who'd been standing on the sidewalk after his car crash, a dozen or more adults of differing ages and dress, sauntering along, smiling and chatting with each other as if on a day out. A few caught his eye and waved at him, though Gray didn't recognise the action as a greeting. It looked more like…, like a rapid one-armed breast stroke, an indication to move aside. A warning! Of what?

Abruptly Gray's world turned red once more, and the words "Late, late," echoed in his mind. Then, just as suddenly, he was peering at the back of a man's jacket receding from the tip of his nose. Alf's extended family had the good manners to step to one side as the man hurried along the path, oblivious to having just passed through Gray's spirit, but aware of the cold shiver which briefly and unaccountably stroked his skin on such a warm day.

Alf caught Gray's arm as he reeled unsteadily. 'Watch where you're going, Dave, I don't think it's polite to go barging through people like that. Besides, it knocks you off balance if you're not careful,' he said with a mocking chortle.

'Yeah, thanks,' Gray mumbled ungratefully, shrugging off the assistance and standing his ground. The unexpected encounter made him angry, and allowing his emotions to show as he had done over the little Asian girl was embarrassing. He was accustomed to being in control for Christ's sake! Of his environment, his life, of other people. This whole thing, whatever it was, verged on madness. He was losing it. Bigtime. 'Listen to me, Alf, and listen good,' he exploded in the tone usually reserved for errant subordinates, particularly trainee surgeons. 'I'm getting more than a little pissed off with all this. Finish it now and take me back. I want this dream, this frigging nightmare, over. Come on, *do it!*'

'Dave, Dave,' Alf said with a shrug, and shook his head sadly. 'I don't know how. I've already told yer, I'm not doing anything apart from stickin' with you. I go where you go.'

'That's not bloody good enough, Alf. You seem to...'

'That is enough gentlemen. I will not put up with you yelling and blaspheming in public like common fishwives. Show a little respect and dignity!' Alf's mother entered the fray from behind.

Both men stood with their heads down; schoolboys in front of the headmistress.

'Mr Gray, I'll thank you for not haranguing my son in such a manner,' she said, scolding, fists on hips. 'He is simply doing the job that was asked of him to the best of his,' she looked Alf up and down, 'rather meagre abilities. If you have any questions regarding the purpose of your..., your excursion, please address them to me now and be done with it. I shall attempt to answer you as best I can, though of course there are limits both to my knowledge and the amount of information I am allowed to impart.'

Chapter 3

'Yes, er, ma'am. Thank you,' Gray stammered, at once contrite. This diminutive woman had all the charisma of a refined and polite sledgehammer. 'I apologise if I've caused any upset either to you or your son,' he tilted his head towards the smirking figure of Alf who was thoroughly enjoying the moment, 'but quite frankly I'm no longer prepared to be a part of all this. Whatever's going on, I want out.'

'Do you indeed?' She regarded Gray implacably. 'It would seem you do not fully comprehend the situation, Mr Gray, nor I suspect, have you even attempted to try. But,' she huffed, 'I suppose one must make allowances. A lot has happened and some confusion is understandable.'

Gray nodded dumbly, inviting her to continue.

'In spite of your undoubted skills as a surgeon and a doctor, it is apparent that over the years you have lost direction, and sadly, a certain degree of futility has crept into your attitude towards work and life. It seems you harbour grave doubts about your continued usefulness to mankind, yet you continue to practise, and more importantly, do so without the passion and compassion that once drove you. You even have the audacity to hold an opinion on whether someone would be better off dead. As Alfred remarked, what gives you that right?'

'You know it wasn't meant that way!'

'Do I? All life is precious to the being which holds it, Mr Gray. Why do you assume my son, or anyone else for that matter, might decline into a miserable and lonely old age? Who are you to judge misery or loneliness? Who are you to pass judgement at all?'

Gray had no answer.

'Quite!' She lowered her eyebrows fractionally. 'All of which brings us to the crux of the matter. Your soul feels broken and betrayed, Mr Gray, and providence has supplied a means by which it might heal itself. It is neither me, nor Alfred, who control the events you are witnessing. Rather, it is your own essence, fighting for its very survival. Consequently, if you wish to terminate this examination of your life and work, if you are no longer prepared to be a party to it, then you must look to yourself, and no other. For only you know the truth which is in your heart, and in the final analysis we are each our own judge and jury. I would, however, give you some advice. Spirits cannot harm you, so let go of your fear and belligerence, and learn from this rare gift you have been granted.'

She turned and walked away, back to the other members of her family, and as Gray watched, they all faded to invisibility.

'See what I mean?' Alf beamed with admiration. 'What a woman! Way over my head though. What about you, Dave, she make any sense to you?'

'A little, I think.' His voice was flat and unsure. He turned to face Alf, 'I'm sorry I lost my temper with you.'

'Don't worry about it old son, you're under a lot of stress. No offence taken. Now, where to next?'

'Not a clue, Alf.'

'Well we'd better make a move soon, I think we've been spotted.' Alf tilted his head and rolled his eyes downwards. Sitting on the grass a few yards away, a Red Setter was staring directly up at both of them, ears cocked, offering a paw and whining for attention.

Instinctively they both searched around for the owner and spotted a man approaching directly from somewhere in the middle of the park. Smartly dressed in a dark pin-striped suit, club tie and white shirt, with a full head of buttery-grey hair which had once been blonde, Gray recognised the resolute stride immediately. There was no doubting it; hooded lids above intelligent eyes, elegant features marred by a rugby-smeared nose, stiff upper lip machine-gun speech.

'How the hell are you, David?' His right hand stretched out in a cheery welcome.

Gray looked as if he'd seen a ghost, which of course he had, but by then he was accustomed to that particular aspect of things and it wasn't the spiritual apparition which unnerved him. The man was Gray's irascible old boss, his final mentor before he himself was appointed a consultant. In spite of emergency surgery, he had died from a bleeding ulcer a few years after retirement. At the time it was big news in the small world of surgery: multi-organ failure with every available specialist pulling out all the stops for a senior colleague. Gray recalled the packed memorial service, nearly twenty years previously.

They shook hands. 'Hello sir, this is an unexpected pleasure.' Which it was. He admired and respected Gerald "Gerry" Westman, both as a man and a surgeon, and knew his prickly nature was mostly a put-on front.

'Please accept my apologies for being late, David. Bit of a cock-up on the communications side I'm afraid. Shit happens wherever you are, believe me, just a question of how one deals with it. Never mind though, caught up with each other in the end, haven't we? He shifted his attention to Alf, introducing himself with a further handshake. 'Gerry Westman, and you are?'

'Alf Angel.'

'Glad to meet you, Alf. Please call me Gerry. Are you coming along too?'

'I'm with Dave all the way, mate. I mean, Gerry.' Alf moved a protective step closer to Gray.

'Excellent,' Westman announced, though he appeared doubtful.

'Er, where are we going?' Gray said.

'Look, I realise what's happened is a bit of a shock to you both, but nonetheless, there are protocols and procedures to follow. So, if you'd care to join me in my office for a few minutes, we can get it all sorted.'

Alf and Gray exchanged a quizzical glance just as the dog's patience finally ran out. It jumped up, eager to be petted and stroked. But was too late. They were already gone.

4

Gerry Westman's "office" was modern and spacious. Floor to ceiling windows made up three walls while the fourth was plain red brickwork decorated with a collection of framed antique prints interspersed with photos of his family. Outside the office and far below, a blanket of cloud spread to the horizon, hiding whatever ground features lay beneath. Above was nothing but endless blue. Like flying over the Atlantic in winter, Gray thought, except there was no sense of movement. It was as if they were in the penthouse of a five-thousand floor office block, though the recessed glass denied any completely vertical examination to confirm the impression.

The room itself was dominated by a long central table made of yew or a wood of similar light texture, its expansive pristine surface gleaming luxuriously in the bright sunlight. Around the table twenty exquisitely carved Louis XIV chairs with gold-leaf marquetry and scarlet padding were arranged in perfect order, and covering the floor a deep fitted carpet mirrored the colour of the cerulean sky. If this was Gerry Westman's office, it obviously doubled as some sort of committee room. Nothing else marred the opulent yet utilitarian space - no phones, no filing cabinets, no computer terminals, and, Gray noted with a little uneasiness, no doors.

Alongside Gray at one of the windows, Alf gave out a low whistle. 'That's quite a view, Gerry.'

Westman stood behind them both, rocking gently on the balls of his feet with a smug grin on his lips. 'It's only the default location, Alf, but I like it. We could have this if you prefer.'

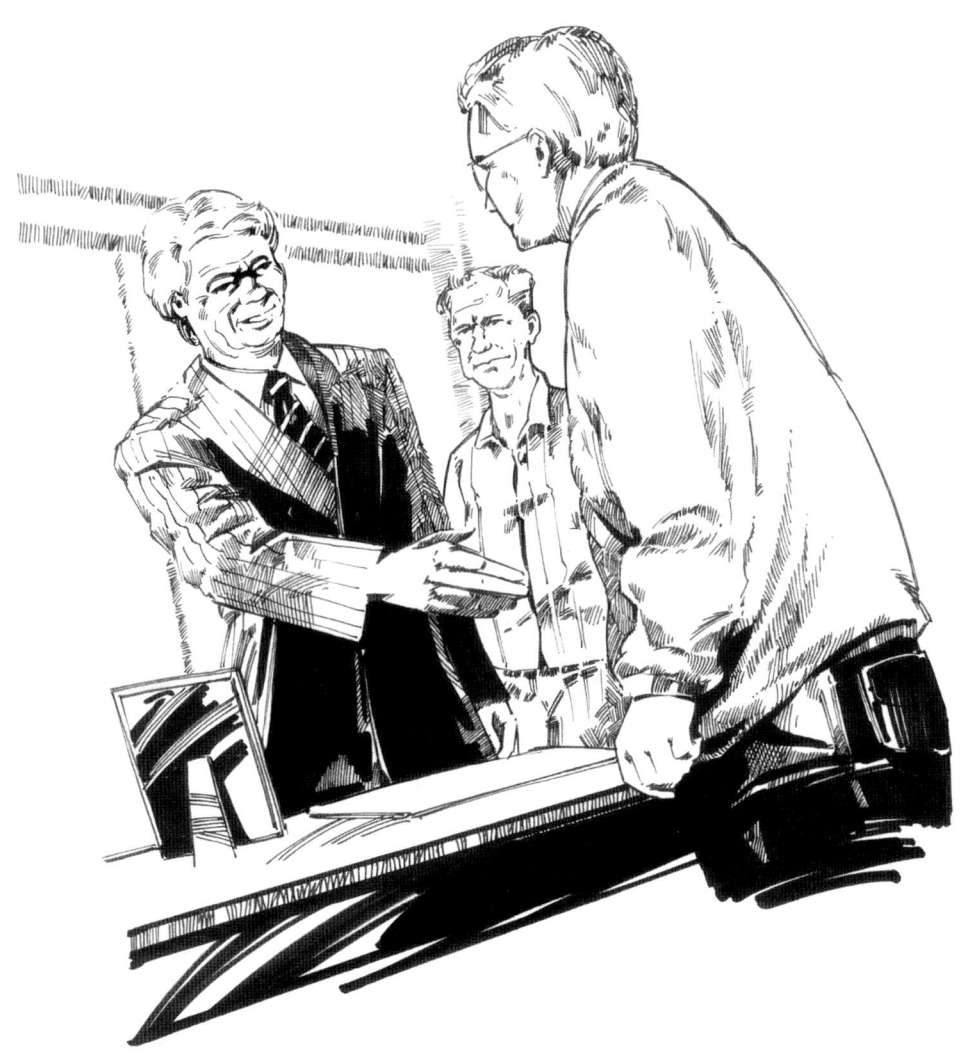

Chapter 4

Through the windows the scene blinked to a deserted tropical beach, complete with palm trees, golden sand and lapping surf.

'Or this.'

They were under the sea watching a coral reef with shoals of brightly coloured tropical fish.

'Or.'

The office was in space, orbiting the Earth.

Alf and Gray instinctively staggered backwards from the window for fear of falling through it, and at once they were in the original penthouse, with clouds, and sky, and rock-steady floor beneath their feet.

'Exactly,' Westman announced. 'We can go wherever we want; New York, Delhi, even Mars if you like. But I find this place the most peaceful and offers fewer distractions when I've business to attend to, except of course when a high-flying jet passes close by, though at this altitude they are, thankfully, few and far between. Now let's take a pew chaps, there's a few formalities to go through.'

Westman pulled out a pen and notebook from the inside pocket of his jacket and led them to one end of the long table where he and Alf took a seat.

'I'd rather stand,' Gray said, hovering with his hands clasping the back of a chair.

'That's okay with me, David.' Westman smiled knowingly and looked up at him. 'Let's start with your details first, shall we? Then I'll do Alf's.'

Gray nodded his assent.

'Mother's full maiden name and year of death.' He held his pen poised over the notebook. 'I presume you'll want to see her.'

He did. More than anything else. 'Veronica Gilbert, twelve years ago, that'll be…'

'Close enough. I'll find her.' He scribbled something down. 'Father?'

Gray squirmed. 'I don't know much about him. His name was Brian, but I never met him. Sorry, that's wrong. What I mean is, I don't remember him. He was in the RAF and died in a plane crash just after the war. There's old photographs of him holding me as a baby, but the sad truth is I wouldn't recognise him unless I had a picture with me.'

'Any siblings?'

'No. Mum never remarried. I was brought up by her and my grandparents.'

Westman scribbled again. 'I can work on that one, no problem. If he's here, he'll be with her. Now, what was your purpose in life, and did you achieve it?'

'Sorry?' Gray said, nonplussed.

'The purpose of your life. What was it?'

'Not a clue. I thought I was here to find out.'

'But you must know!' Westman sounded and looked astonished. 'How can you have died and not know your purpose?'

'But I'm not dead.' Gray's face betrayed his own incomprehension. 'Is that what you think?'

Westman snapped the notebook shut and glanced at Alf, who shook his head, eyes down.

'Well, when are you due to die?'

'I don't know,' Gray explained. 'I thought I already had, but Alf here,' he pointed, 'tells me I haven't. And so does his mother, of all people.'

Westman's mouth opened and closed several times, but no words came. He hurriedly replaced the pen and notebook in his pocket, rested both hands gently and carefully on the table in front of him, took a deep breath, exhaled slowly, and then lifted his eyes to Gray's. 'David, are you absolutely, one hundred percent, sure you are not dead?'

Gray felt anger and frustration stir in his chest. 'I don't know, do I!' He spat the words out. 'I'd have thought it's you who should be telling me!'

Westman ignored Gray's outburst and turned calmly towards Alf. 'How about you?'

Alf was clearly enjoying the confusion they were causing. He shook his head with a broad smile, 'Nah, Gerry. Not yet.'

With the swift precise movements of a man who'd come to an uncertain decision, Westman suddenly stood up. 'Please wait here, gentlemen. I'll be back shortly.' Then he turned and strode towards the centre of the brick wall, passing through it without faltering.

Leaning back in his chair, Alf cackled loudly. 'Well, Dave, looks like we've thrown a bleedin' big spanner in the works somewhere, whadyereckon? Good fun though, ain't it?'

Gray sighed to himself as a maelstrom of ambiguous bewilderment churned in his mind. No, it wasn't fun. Anything but. Distracted by his thoughts, he began wandering the perimeter of the room, idly tapping the knuckles of his right hand on the glass of the windows and the bricks of the wall as he went. It was a habit developed through years of treading long hospital corridors while seeking solace and solutions for problematic patients. Tap, tap; tub, tub; tap, tap; tub, tub. The noise was soothing and helped his concentration; tap, tap… Then, with an unexpected jolt, he realised everything was solid. It felt hard and natural against the skin of his fingers; it made a noise! Experimenting further, he shoved hard against the brickwork, but couldn't push his hand through. With no door to be seen anywhere, he reached the obvious conclusion. 'Alf, I think we're locked in!'

'Course we are. They ain't going to let us wander around heaven on our own, are they? Gerry thought we were dead, but we're not, so he's gone off to check on what to do next. He'll be back soon.'

Gray passed his gaze over the wall, searching the length and breadth of it with awe. Then he patted and stroked it. 'Do you really think heaven's on the other side of this?'

'It's just a name, Dave. I think there's got to be lots of heavens, 'cos my heaven wouldn't be the same as yours or anyone else's, would it?' Alf reasoned. He sat with his hands clasped behind his head, legs stretched out and bare feet crossed at the ankles; a picture of nonchalant contentment. 'Mine would be quiet and peaceful, with a few old friends to keep me company and a bit o' general construction work to keep me interested. Nothing too heavy though; joinery or plastering, something like that. Oh yeah, and tea. There'd have to be tea, huge steaming mugs of the stuff whenever you wanted, thick with sugar and condensed milk. It wouldn't be heaven otherwise, would it? Not for me at any rate.' The vision made Gray hoot with laughter, which was Alf's primary intention. Then he changed the subject, gently. 'Dave, I'm sorry to hear yer dad died when you were so young. What was it like, growing up without a father?'

'Didn't know any different, Alf. Might as well ask you the same question. What was it like for you without a mother?'

'I asked first.' He leaned forward, elbows on the table. 'Come on, we've nothing better to do.'

'Well, like I said, I was young and didn't know any better.' Gray began circuiting the room again, remembering. 'Mum moved back to Yorkshire to live with her parents after she was widowed, so I grew up with her and my grandparents in a rambling old place in the country. I thought it was brilliant, a huge playground just for me, but I suppose it was lonely with no other children in the house. And as I got older I think I did develop some resentment when my friends talked about their dads or their brothers and sisters, but at the same time I felt sorry for mum who had no man in her life except me. Eventually my grandfather persuaded her to send me to boarding school so I could be with other kids and develop normally. It was the right decision for me, but it broke her heart, even though I was home most weekends and all the holidays. Seems I've spent most of my life worried about her being sad and lonely and hoping she'd find someone else to fall in love with.' He sighed. 'In the end she never did.'

'If you'd had a father, you wouldn't be the caring man you are,' Alf stated in an assured, matter-of-fact tone. 'You'd probably be a completely different person.'

Gray stopped pacing. Is that how others saw him? Was he a caring man? All he knew was that he didn't feel like one. And hadn't done for years.

Westman marched back through the wall like a whirlwind laced with venomous wrath, his entrance so startling even laid-back Alf jumped to his feet. 'Right chaps, I've been making a few enquiries,' he said through clenched teeth.

Gray smiled to himself, recalling what form Gerry Westman's enquiries usually took. Someone, somewhere, had just had the biggest carpeting of their life; or should that be death?

'David, I understand you're not dead, and what's more, you're suffering from a touch of burn-out.'

'Am I?'

'Don't deny it, David, you're only deluding yourself. I know what's in your soul and it's now clear why I've been recruited. I thought I'd taught you well, but it seems there's a few things I overlooked. We need to finish the job.' Westman pointed a finger at the brick wall. 'Look.'

It had changed to a cinema screen, and on it a young Gray was operating. Alf was enthralled.

'Do you remember that operation, David?' Westman said.

Gray shook his head. 'Looks like an appendix.'

'It's the first one you ever did on your own. The registrar is watching TV in the mess. He trusted you enough to leave you to do it alone because you had good hands.'

'So what?' Gray said.

'I want you to recall your feelings.'

Gray stared at the screen, watching himself working. The image seemed to act as some form of sensorial magnifier, for his mind stretched out of control back to an operation he couldn't even remember doing. There must have been tens of thousands between then and the present - most were forgotten, and any feelings he had for them lost or hidden in his psyche - but he found himself being deluged in a torrent of emotions from thirty-five years in the past. They washed over and through him in waves of goosebumps; trepidation, happiness, elation, fulfillment, wonderment; and all stemming from a simple appendix operation. Yet at the same time, he knew he'd arrived home. He could do this. It was easy. He'd been born to it.

Then the screen changed to a few days later with Gray standing by a fifteen year old boy lying in hospital bed, checking the temperature chart, and telling him he could go home. With his own hands he had cured this young lad, watched him recover, ran to his bedside three times a day, just to make sure. With his own hands! It was magic. Pure magic.

Gray staggered at the intensity of the sensation, and then it was gone.

'You had it once, David,' Westman said, almost goading. 'Let's go see if we can find it again.'

ooooooooooooooooooooooooooooooooo

It was an operating amphitheatre, the likes of which Gray had only seen in old paintings and prints. They were on the "stage", an area of wooden floor no more than ten paces wide and covered in a light sprinkling of sawdust. In the middle stood a large and heavy table the size of a waist-high single bed and constructed of smoothly sanded timber. It resembled a huge butcher's block, save for a number of thick leather straps attached down each side. Above the table hung an elaborate array of burning oil lamps and reflecting mirrors, and rising away from the stage, steeply terraced ranks of benches were fashioned in a semi-circle, enough to seat maybe fifty on-lookers. The room was clad in panelled oak and well lit through high leaded windows, and adorning the walls were oil-painted portraits of past luminaries.

Blinking in surprise, Gray and Alf looked around as Westman answered their unspoken question. 'Saint Bartholomew's hospital, about 1820. I thought we might benefit from seeing what surgery was like then.'

As he spoke, a crowd of young men in double-breasted tailcoats entered noisily through the tall wide doors and proceeded to occupy the benches. They were followed by a more senior man with thinning white hair and large mutton-chop whiskers. Positioning himself behind the butcher's block, he rested his hands and leaned on it like an orator waiting for the excited hum of the audience to settle down.

This must be the surgeon, Gray decided, wondering who exactly it was.

'John Abernethy, Professor of Surgery,' Westman continued his commentary.

The three were standing out of the way in one corner of the stage. Alf seemed mightily impressed, 'Blimey, a professor!'

'Gentlemen,' Abernethy began in a bored monotone. 'The patient fell from his horse last week and sustained a compound fracture of the right lower tibia and fibula. A Pott's fracture, named after Sir Percival Pott, the distinguished barber-surgeon who once graced this institution with his considerable talent, and had the misfortune to suffer the same injury. Miasma has taken hold in the patient's wound, as is natural, and amputation is required. By God's will, he may live thereafter, but without surgery he will surely die.'

'Did he say something about a barber?' Alf said, as if his ears were playing up.

'All surge...' Gray and Westman started speaking simultaneously, before Gray conceded to his senior colleague.

'All surgeons,' Westman began again, with a gracious nod to Gray, 'were originally barbers. Not only did they cut hair, but traditionally they also lanced abscesses and boils, dressed wounds, pulled teeth, and whatever else they were capable of. Some even developed particular skills removing bladder stones or setting broken bones. That's why a barber's pole is red and white, to signify blood and bandages. Henry the Eighth recognised the Barber-Surgeons Company three hundred years ago, back in 1540.' He pointed to a huge painting which had pride of place on one of the walls. 'That's him up there, giving the royal charter to the first master surgeon, a chap by the name of Vicary.'

Alf whistled through his teeth. 'You boys go back some way then, Gerry.'

Westman smiled. 'Yes, Alf, English surgery has a long and honourable history, but through all the centuries, physicians would never recognise us as proper doctors. That's why we're all called "mister", and Mr David Gray here is part of that tradition.' He dropped his voice and winked, 'I'm hoping our trip here might inspire him.'

'I doubt this could inspire anyone,' Gray murmured with distaste, indicating the entrance doors.

Four assistants carried the patient in on a stretcher and quickly placed him upon the table. The man was in a wretched state; filthy nightshirt, matted hair, glistening with feverish sweat and rambling incoherently. Abernethy stood back, removed his tailcoat and handed it to one of the assistants. The other three busied themselves with the leather bindings, positioning and restraining the man according to Abernethy's instructions, leaving both legs hanging over the end of table. The right foot, swollen blue-black with gangrene, hung limply from the calf at an odd angle, attached only by muscle, skin and sinew. A ragged wound ran across the shin, shining scarlet with infection and baring the white bone beneath. It bubbled and dripped a mixture of green pus and blood as the leg swung loosely, and the stench caused the first few rows of students to lift scented handkerchiefs to their noses. The good left ankle was strapped to the table leg.

Abernethy rolled up his sleeves and straightened his waistcoat while the brawny assistants, clearly men of some experience, took their positions. One put a tanned-hide pillow over the patient's face and held on tight, as if attempting to smother him. Another, the biggest, lay over the chest and belly as a physical restraint while the remaining two helped the surgeon. It was all done with the speed and precision of a planned, well-rehearsed ambush, with few words exchanged.

A slip-knot tourniquet cord was tightened around the upper thigh as Abernethy picked out an instrument from the mahogany box presented to him. He chose what looked like a two foot carving knife with a curved blade and black ebony handle. Then the leg was held out and he started cutting, just above the knee, swift deft strokes down to bone. The muffled screams from beneath the pillow were piteous, but the surgery continued in a frenzy of glinting steel and gushing blood. One of the assistants kicked a wooden bucket into place to catch the spill.

Alf gasped. 'Ain't they goin' to put him to sleep?'

'No,' Gray explained, his eyes fixed on the operation. 'Anaesthesia hasn't been discovered yet. He might be drunk on gin if somebody was kind enough to supply it, and if he's really lucky, he might have had a slug of laudanum. But that's it. Nothing else is available. The idea of the pillow, apart from stifling the noise, is to cause a degree of suffocation and unconsciousness. Got to get it right though. Obviously.'

As they watched the pillow was lifted clear. The man's face was a mottled purple, and he sucked in great heaving gasps of air before the pillow descended once more, and the muffled screams continued.

'I once knew an anaesthetist like that,' Westman observed drily.

By then Abernethy was sawing, a fierce concentration on his features, and beads of sweat on his brow.

'This is terrible Dave. They're killin' 'im.'

'This Alf,' Westman said, 'is the height of sophisticated surgery. Yet David here, thinks the work he does is primitive! By comparison he's a miracle worker.'

'Is he going to cauterise the stump?' Gray said, ignoring his boss's jibe.

'No, they're long past that by now. See, he's using linen thread to tie the vessels, but he'll leave the ends long so they hang out of the wound and fall out on their own in a week or two.'

'He hasn't a cat in hell's chance of surviving long enough for that. You know it.'

'Hey guys. I'm 'ere too, remember. What are you talkin' about?'

'That man, Alf, that poor bastard screaming there on the table,' Gray said, emphasizing the point for Westman's benefit, 'has about a ten percent chance of surviving. And even if he does, with one leg how's he going to earn a living in this Godforsaken age? He can't exactly go on the social, can he?'

Two minutes after starting, Abernethy finished to a round of applause and washed his bare hands in a bucket of soapy water. The patient, mercifully, had lapsed into a state of fitful unconsciousness brought on by pain, the shock of blood loss, and septicaemia. The assistants busied themselves loosing the leather bindings and dressing the amputation stump in oiled cloths to keep it air tight, thereby preventing the ingress of further "miasma".

Gray snorted in derision.

'Don't be so judgmental, David,' Westman reprimanded his pupil. 'You've a bad habit of that. Abernethy is doing his best. They're all doing their best with the knowledge available to them. Just as I did. Just as you do. He believes air corrupts wounds, it's the accepted wisdom of the day. So what? That doesn't make him heartless, otherwise he wouldn't be here. This is a charitable institute.'

'Don't he get paid then?'

'No, Alf. He earns money by treating well-to-do clients in their homes, or teaching surgery and anatomy to a few apprentices, or dressers, as you've just witnessed. They pay to work with him. This evening he's back here dissecting a corpse for the benefit of these same students,' Westman waved a hand at the emptying ranks of seats, 'who pay an admission fee for the privilege.'

'And he'll be doing it on the same table, no doubt,' Gray added, mindful of the woeful ignorance of hygiene and infection.

'Hey, Gerry, that sounds like Burke and Hare stuff, murders and grave robbing an' all!'

'Actually, you're not far off the mark, Alf, but those two were in Edinburgh before proper laws were enforced. Most corpses are executed criminals, and having your body donated to science is part of the death-sentence.'

With the patient carried out and the students gone, Abernethy was left standing alone in the empty theatre. He rolled his sleeves down to his wrists with a slow deliberation, shrugged on his tailcoat with an audible sigh, and then stood for a moment in quiet contemplation. Rain clouds had gathered outside, darkening the room, and light from the oil lamps overhead cast gloomy shadows across the bloodied sawdust on the floor. Abernethy looked down at the damning evidence, then cast his eyes heavenwards.

'If it please you, Lord,' he prayed aloud, 'allow your divine intervention to shine on my labours, and forgive me the suffering I have inflicted this day. By your grace and providence, may he live.' Then he turned and shuffled out.

Westman took it as his cue. 'That man cares, David. In spite of the appalling death rate, the infection which he doesn't comprehend, the pain he causes, the screams of his patients, he cares deeply for human life, and you have the gall to scoff and criticise his efforts. Yet you are a product of his learning and teaching, and in a very real sense he is one of your forefathers. He and thousands more like him who had the guts to carry on, against the odds, the disappointments, and the self-doubt. And all this was only three or four lifetimes before your high-tech operation on Alf using electricity, anaesthesia, antibiotics, and whatever else Abernethy would give his eye teeth for. You function as well as you do because of the research and the courage of men like him.'

'I know,' Gray said, his mood sullen and brooding. 'But you don't understand how I feel.'

'Well tell us then! We're all ears, aren't we, Alf?'

Alf nodded enthusiastically. 'Yeah, come on, Dave, spill the beans.'

'The fire's gone sir.'

'David, I think we're both familiar enough with each other to be on first name terms, don't you? Call me Gerry.'

'I'm sorry, Gerry.'

'That's better. Makes me feel more at ease too. Nobody's called me "sir" since before I died.' Westman smiled at his old pupil, a natural paternalistic gesture, for that is how he felt.

'The fire's gone out of me, Gerry. And I don't know how, or why, or when. I still care, honestly I do. But... Oh, where do I start?' Gray stomped around and waved his arms fretfully, frustrated to distraction by his inability to bare his feelings. Held in check for so many years, submerged so deeply and buried so well, it was painful to dig them up for inspection. All he could find in the first shovel-full was blind anger.

'Alf here,' he hissed, pointing malevolently, 'has just shown me the first two patients who ever made me think about how useless I am. How pointless this whole damned business is. They all die, Gerry. Get it yet? You of all people should know that. We all die, so what's the point of it all? I could do more for mankind by being a sanitary engineer. Fresh water and safe sewage for the whole world! Do you realise half the population who ever lived on Earth died of malaria? And that's ever, Gerry. Repeat, *ever!* And what have I spent my life doing? Giving old men like Alf here,' he jabbed his finger again, 'a few more years of living so they can go on to die of cancer or something worse. Or fixing varicose veins and lumps and bumps for cosmetic reasons. So I suppose that's it. All doctors, including me, would be better off as plumbers with a syringe full of morphine in our back pockets. We'd do more good providing clean water and pain-killers to everyone. Direct, simple, obvious!'

'Dave, Dave. It's nothing to do with me! How many times do I have to say it? I'm just along for the ride, to look afte...'

'Excuse me, Alf, I apologise for interrupting, but I think we have a serious problem here.' Westman observed Gray with a furrowed brow and pursed lips. The old chief was concerned. Deeply. He recognised the symptoms. This was not an act. His charge was in dire trouble. 'David, old chap. You're not the first, or the last, to think the same. Believe me, I've been down that road myself. You still care, as you have so eloquently explained.' Westman flashed a false smile. 'But it's conceited to think you're the only one who's ever reached this impasse. Granted, you've arrived there while you're still alive, but then again, you've always been precocious. The problem is, you're not supposed to be feeling this way for a long time yet, when you will hopefully, like me, be invited to join the Dead Medics' Society.'

But Gray was on a mad roll, deaf to anyone but himself. 'I'm not interested, Gerry. I'm already in every damned society going. Royal Society of Medicine, the College, the Vascular Surgeons, oncology groups, committees for this and that, even the wimpy paediatrician lot. They're all the same; prattling on about a six-month survival benefit for this chemotherapy or that operation, when half the world still needs fresh water! Why can't they see it, the plumbing thing, the madness of it all?'

Westman took a seat on the front row of the theatre before answering, coolly crossing his legs and brushing imaginary dust from the knees of his immaculate trousers. 'We all feel the same way, David.'

Chapter 4

'Who do?'

'Dead Medics. We all feel the same, even Lister. He was the founding member.'

'You've met Lister?' Gray said incredulously.

'I've met them all, David. And believe it or not, they're quite impressed by my own meagre contributions. Research, publications, teaching. That type of thing.'

'They know about them?'

'Of course they do. They're the inspiration in all of us. Why would anyone do medical research if it weren't for the muse, the insight, the revelation? It's certainly not for the money is it? And once finished, wouldn't the instigator want to check on the results? See it's been done right, reported correctly? Natural isn't it?'

'You mean the likes of Lister are still working?'

'And Fleming, and Barnard, and all the others. But working's not quite the right expression. We have lots of ideas but all we can do is try to get them across. After all, none of us can still seed a Petri dish with bacteria or wield a scalpel can we?' Westman suddenly chuckled to himself.

'What's so funny?'

'Petri. He gets quite worked up about it. Never was keen on Germans myself. Too…,' Westman scratched his chin, searching for the word, 'too Teutonic. Desperate for total control. Keeps trying to organise us into chapters and gets furious when he can't get his thoughts through to whichever mortal he's trying to influence.'

'For God's sake, Gerry. What are you talking about?'

Alf, feeling out of it, and possibly intimidated by the two doctors talking "over his head", wandered off to examine the portraits on the walls in greater detail.

'Dead medics, David. When you die, you will doubtless want to join the DMS. In fact, yes that's it, I'll nominate you.' Westman observed his junior colleague thoughtfully, 'But who shall we get as a second?'

'Gerry, listen to me. I'm at a loss to know what's going on right here, right now. And I'm certainly not interested in joining some Dead Medics' Society, no matter who proposes me.'

Westman sat up straight on the bench and looked around. Alf was many yards away, closely inspecting Holbein's painting of Henry VIII, and out of earshot.

'David,' he said, deadly serious. 'I know your secret. You have compassion failure. That's very serious for a doctor of any sort, but normally it comes *after* death, when one realises death is simply a transition, not the end of existence. That's when a doctor questions the purpose of his calling and concludes it's all been a waste of time. But for you those doubts seem to have come early, and without the support of colleagues who understand it's a very serious malady. It may even lead to suicide. When I died I was taken on much the same trip you are now on, and for much the same reasons. But the point is, David, it was after my transition, not before, and I had friends, other doctors, who helped me to see my truth. Somehow, you've come to appreciate death isn't the end while you are still alive. How did you do it?'

'Don't really know, Gerry. It just crept over me.' He hesitated, 'Not in a religious way though, I can't stand that nonsense.'

'I know that.' Westman gestured impatiently, urging Gray to continue.

'Well, it's obvious really. Conservation of energy sort of thing. The spark of life is energy, so it can't be snuffed out can it? And you're living proof, if living's the right word.'

'Quite so.' Westman shook his head, saddened at the consequences of his pupil's knowledge. 'So now, in your unguided disenchanted way, you've lost the drive and the passion. The fire as you call it. You exist as an unfeeling processor of information fed to you, and out comes the processed equation, the optimal path to take to prolong a patient's life because that's what's expected and it's scientific and you can't be challenged or criticised by your peers for the decision you've made. And the sisters and brothers, the daughters and sons, the husbands and wives, the mothers and fathers, all want their loved one to live longer because that's what's expected of them. But in reality they're all scared of facing either the decision or the whole process of a relative dying, and want someone else to make it all go away. And you're sick of their cowardice and their transference of blame and guilt because they never cared for their "loved one" in the first place. And they don't understand death doesn't matter because no-one really dies, but even if you told them they wouldn't believe you anyway. And you plod on thinking it's all pointless but doing everything properly just so you can't be accused of negligence and are able to say, "We've done all we can, but...". Am I right David? Is that what you're going through?'

The knot in Gray's throat wouldn't allow him to speak, so he nodded instead, and tried to hide the grateful tear in his eye.

'Compassion failure! I knew it!' Westman stood up and called to the far end of the room. 'Come along, Alf, there's work to do.'

5

Gray was becoming accustomed to out-of-body travel; a feathery whoosh in his chest, a momentary change in texture of the light, often with some blurred out-of-focus images of people and things - streets, trees, the sea, clouds - and then everything back in clear focus again.

It was another operating theatre, though more recognisable than the last: green tiled walls and floor, a sink for washing, no auditorium, and the butcher's block replaced by a padded leather table.

A woman was lying on it, asleep, courtesy of a youthful looking man in a brown dress suit. Over her mouth and nose he held a leather mask attached by canvas elephant tubing to a glass bottle half-filled with clear fluid. Apart from her head and left breast, she was covered in wet towels. The breast was being removed.

The surgeon also wore a dress suit, though the felt collar was turned up and the sleeves rolled back, revealing muscular forearms and bloody bare hands. Two male assistants were similarly attired and bloodied. A few feet away stood what looked like a camera tripod, but the copper device mounted on top was not for photographs. A third assistant pumped continuously at a wooden handle attached to the machine, and from its spout a mist of hissing spray emerged in clouds, drenching the operating field, the table, and the surgeon's arms.

'King's College Hospital, late 1870s,' Westman announced to Gray and Alf. 'I want you to meet this man, David. Let's get closer so we can watch him work.' Thoughtfully he turned to Alf, 'Are you alright with this? Not squeamish?'

Alf smiled sheepishly. 'If it's all the same to you, Gerry, and I don't want to be disrespectful or nothing, but I think I'll just stand by the window in the corner till you two gents are ready. See what the view's like in, what year did you say?'

'About 1878.' Westman grinned and slapped Alf on the back as he sauntered away, still in bare feet and pyjamas. 'We won't keep you waiting long.'

The surgeon was meticulous and speedy, and when Westman and Gray approached near enough to see, it was clear his collar was turned up to stop the spray dripping down his neck or sousing his rampant sideburns.

'Ether?' Gray nodded toward the anaesthetist.

'Chloroform,' Westman answered. 'And look, he's tying off the vessels with sterilised catgut and cutting the sutures short, not leaving them long to fall out later. And the instruments are solid steel, no filthy wooden handles.'

'The carbolic spray machine, a Lister donkey to disinfect the air?'

'Yes. This is the era of antiseptic surgery, less than twenty years since Louis Pasteur proved the existence of bacteria and rang the death knell on miasma, or air souring wounds. Of course, in another twenty years or so there'll be aseptic surgery and this will all be gone, replaced with sterile gowns and gloves and masks.'

Gray studied the operation. The surgeon was slick, quick, and knew his anatomy. The cancerous breast had already gone - thrown into a metal bucket on the floor - and now he was dissecting the glands from around the arteries, veins and nerves in the armpit.

'Let him finish this tricky bit, then he'll have a chat with us,' Westman announced calmly.

'Okay,' Gray said absently, preoccupied with watching the surgery. He noticed with disapproval the pectoral muscles had been divided to gain better access to the deep tissues - disfiguring and disabling, and only one step removed from excising the muscle completely. Eventually the dissection finished and the surgeon began sewing the skin together over the huge wound.

Chapter 5

Gray recognised the all-too-familiar tension waning in the stance of the man; shoulders drooping, neck relaxing, breathing less rapid, hands working automatically. The end of a successful operation without complication or reason for concern.

As he looked on, the outline of the surgeon blurred, and for a split second Gray thought he was seeing double. Perhaps it was the mist of carbolic spray, the light diffracting through the cloud of droplets and playing tricks? Then, in one quick movement, the surgeon stepped back from the operating table, and at once Gray knew it was no trick of the light. It was as if the man had moved outside of his body in one rearward stride. The flesh continued operating, but the spirit turned and covered the few steps towards Westman.

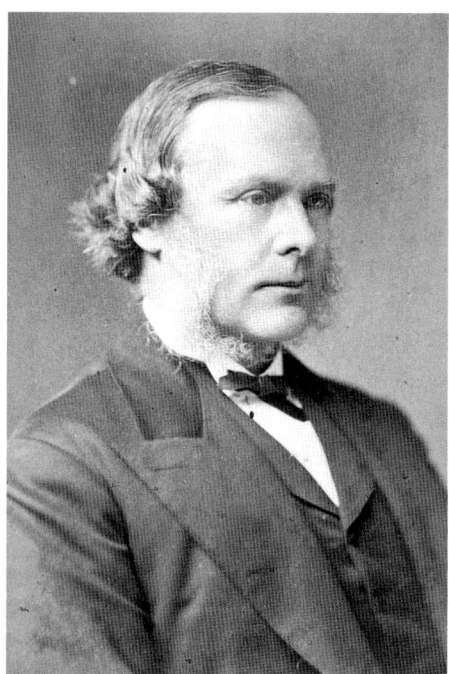

Joseph Lister

Wellcome Library, London

'Greetings, Gerald,' he said, the accent uncultured and vaguely Scottish.

'Hello, Joseph,' Westman said with a wry smile. 'Enjoying yourself?'

The spirit glanced back over his shoulder; his body was still busy sewing up. 'From time to time it's good to feel maself working again.' He turned to face Westman once more. 'Though as I'm sure tha' knows, Gerald,' he grinned, 'the déjà vu can be mighty confusing for a soul until one learns to control the memory. Now, how can I help ye?'

Westman held his arm out towards Gray. 'David, I'd like you to meet Joseph Lister, president and founder member of the Dead Medics' Society. Joseph, this is David Gray.'

Gray, slack jawed, held his hand out and felt it being pumped. 'This is a great honour, sir,' he stuttered.

Joseph Lister! Arguably the most famous surgeon in modern history. The man who convinced the medical world that germs were a fact, and needed to be eliminated from surgical wounds. Pilloried and ridiculed by his peers for introducing antiseptics and operating in a stinking cloud of acrid carbolic, deemed criminally negligent for daring to perform open surgery on broken bones, and then acclaimed internationally for his startling results. His patients lived, their bones mended, wounds healed, and all without the curse of infection.

'Thou's too kind sir, the honour is entirely mine.' Lister bowed and released Gray's hand.

An awkward silence prevailed, hewn from the mute chasm of a century or more between the two. And anyway, what do you say to an icon of his age who died before you were even born?

Westman came to the rescue. 'We were watching you operate Joseph. Most impressive!'

'Yes,' Gray chipped in. 'Beautiful work, Mr Lister.'

'I would ask you not to be quite so deferential, sir.' Lister puffed out, his high starched shirt collar and bow tie momentarily disappearing beneath the whiskered jowls. 'I am quite aware she will not benefit greatly from my ministrations. In fact, she will perish within a few years from bone and brain metastases and I will be heartbroken, for she is my own dearly beloved sister. Still, at least I disallowed the development of a malignant eruption on her chest wall as the cancer consumed the breast, and for that we were both grateful.'

Wide-eyed, Gray glanced toward the woman on the table: a mastectomy on his own sister!

'Sir, ye regard my work here as retarded,' Lister continued. 'And I agree. It is. But at the time it was the best I could muster. Remember, I endured a terrible period when half of all my patients died o' gangrene, and a surgical ward was a stinking charnel house full o' wretches with festering wounds caused by "hospital fever". Many still are, though the general ignorance of such matters is speedily abating. As for treating my own flesh and blood, I couldna' entrust her into the hands of any other because my conscience would not allow it. I came to London from Edinburgh for the express purpose of introducing antisepsis, but colleagues in the English College are proud and stubborn, and presently see no advantage in my methods. Even my fellow surgeons here in King's have yet to be convinced that wee microscopic animals are capable of so much harm.' He sighed heavily, recalling the scorn and derision heaped upon "the man from a provincial Scottish school". 'It was a hard task, but one I invited upon myself, so I perservered with it.'

'You were a brave man, sir,' Gray said, feeling genuinely contrite and humbled, but confused by the tenses Lister used: are we here and now, or then and there?

'No, not brave. I was never brave, but the patients were. Brave as lions, all of them. Don't forget, I've seen and done my fair share of surgery without the wonder of Yankee anaesthesia, and I tell ye now, the screams are heart-breaking. So, compassion yes, God-fearing yes. But never brave.'

'But they died in droves, Mr Lister. How did you, how did any of you, find the courage to carry on?'

'The patients had no choice. Suffer pain or death, or beseech us to operate in spite of the agony and risks. No courage, sir, no bravery, just learning, skill and compassion. Aye, and a fair degree of self-doubt.'

'It's never changed David,' Westman added. 'The science got better, that's all. Thanks to Joseph here, and men like him.'

'But all my patients expect miracles,' Gray pleaded. 'No infection, no pain, no complications. No death even. And if anything does go wrong, it's either my fault or someone else's. Never nature taking its own course.'

Lister laughed out loud. 'My dear man, surgeons have been burned at the stake or had their hands cut off for failing to effect a cure, so your travails are trivial by comparison. In a few years I will be asked to drain an abscess in the armpit of Queen Victoria herself. It will not be a comfortable experience for me, but I will counsel her appropriately as to the risks, and then, not shirking my responsibility, and with care and compassion, I'll put my reputation and the reputation of all my fellow surgeons to the test. That is our lot, every time we put knife to skin. Accept it.'

'David, David,' Westman intoned gently, 'everyone expects miracles when they don't perceive life itself as one. That is the tragedy of the human condition. And some of the sadness and frustration you feel. Isn't it?'

Gray frowned at the impossible situation he found himself in - surely it must be a dream? How could Westman know how he felt? Yes, he was frustrated by the sad decaying emptiness he couldn't shift, an emptiness which had wormed its way into his soul over the years and sapped his love for the job. Yet these two men before him, these surgeons who were long dead, still retained their vigour and enthusiasm but had undergone - how did his old boss put it - the transition. They were aware death in the physical sense was not the end, and that living, as most people understand it, isn't the precious be-all and end-all of existence, but they still had compassion. How was that?

'What exactly is compassion?' Gray blurted out to both of them.

'Sympathetic pity and concern for the sufferings or misfortunes of others,' Lister answered spontaneously with a knowing smile. 'I've been asked that before. Many times in fact. It's from the latin "to suffer with".'

'It's why you're here, it's why we're all here,' Westman added, waving his arms expansively. Alf, still absorbed by the view through the corner window, was included in the gesture. 'We are suffering with you, David. That's the purpose of the Dead Medics' Society. Why Joseph founded it.'

'Go on,' Gray said, hoping for some answers.

Westman began pacing, like he always did when teaching or lecturing, choosing his words carefully. 'Men and women who have devoted themselves to saving the lives of others suddenly discover by their own death that no-one ever dies. This comes as a great shock, and being scientifically inclined, they naturally question and analyse the purpose of their calling. Usually this starts with recounting all the pain they've inflicted in the name of medicine or

Chapter 5

surgery, and finishes with the conclusion it was not only unnecessary, but unnecessarily cruel. Then they bemoan all the sleepless nights, the stolen time and the agonizing soul-searching they themselves went through when a patient died. "For what?" they say. "Here we all are, dead but still alive, so why was I bothering? What was the point?".'

'Exactly,' Gray agreed, nodding his head eagerly; an explanation at last!

Lister narrowed his eyes. He'd been here before, and knew what was coming next.

Westman stopped pacing as he approached the climax of his thesis. 'Corporeal death, as I have told you, is simply a transition. Much as birth is. Nor is death to be fought against tooth and nail like an enemy. Because David, you can't beat it. Everybody dies.'

Alf, who had been listening to the lecture from his window position, marched over towards Westman, his tone and body language unmistakeable: he was furious. 'Fer God's sake, Gerry. Tell him something he doesn't already know. The man's drownin' in doubt, can't yer see that? He wants to know what the bleedin' 'ell he's been up to all these years. And fer that matter, so do I!'

'Whoa, Alf.' Westman put up his hands in self-defence. 'I'm getting towards that, give me some credence!'

'Some what?' Alf spat the words, his right fist clenched jaw high.

Westman blushed and bowed his head. 'Belief, Alf. Believe in me. I've been through it. Honestly I have!'

Alf slowly lowered his sledge-hammer fist and looked towards Gray, who nodded his assent. Then he stood back and took his stance; the pyjama man, a bouncer at the door of knowledge.

Westman adjusted his tie self-consciously, one eye on Alf standing menacingly by his side, and cleared his throat with a brief dry cough. 'The thing is, David, the thing is each of us has to reach our own conclusions. I'm not allowed to tell you mine otherwise you might adopt them for your own eternity, and that wouldn't be fair. Likewise even Lord Lister here...,' he stumbled, 'I'm sorry, Joseph, force of habit. I realise you haven't received that acclamation yet.' He turned his attention back to Gray. 'Even Joseph cannot tell you the answer to your problem.

'Your compassion has flown the nest because you realise the spirit lives on. So what then is your impetus to continue? If it's any comfort, you are not alone. From professors through to general practitioners, we've all pondered the same question, and we've all discovered the answer. Once you reach the solution which makes sense to you, you'll be satisfied and your soul will be calmer, though never totally fulfilled, because the nature of the human spirit is to speculate and wonder. It is your own questioning spirit that has brought you prematurely to this particular situation, which as far as I know, is unique.' A glance at Lister produced a supportive nod of confirmation, so Westman continued. 'You, David, are still alive in body so we cannot be completely candid, but I can tell you this. If you come to the same conclusion the other Dead Medics have reached, as I hope you will and should, you will spend the rest of your life a happy man.'

'Bloody useless then, both of you,' Alf yelled, glaring at Westman and Lister.

'Cool it, Alf,' Gray said. 'They're doing their best.'

'Well it's not good enough, is it? We're here for answers and we ain't getting none. I'm with you through thick and thin, Dave, I promised me ma that, and I'd back her in front of these two any day.'

'Alf, enough! Forget it!'

In the charged stillness that followed Gray's outburst, Lister gave out a magnanimous smile and raised his hands theatrically to his lapels, grabbing each in a fist. The gesture was clearly a preamble and immediately he had his audience's undivided attention, though he addressed only Gray. 'I founded the DMS exactly because of the torment you are undergoing, Mr Gray. Medicine, after all, is a vocation, a calling to help one's fellow man which can seldom be denied. You are born with it, live with it, and die with it. And even after death the siren still sings her song for me and others like me, as it surely will for you. Because laddie, and mark this well, that calling spirit is part of your soul,

Chapter 5

immutable and everlasting. So what then can we do? Ignore it and allow ourselves to wither like a plant denied sustenance, or satisfy the yearning, the need to care? There can only be one way, and that is the prime function of the Dead Medics' Society; to support and sustain our fellow souls. For we each know and understand how great a burden is the need to care, and how impossible it is to discard that load.

'You want answers, Mr Gray. I assure you, sir, that neither Gerald or myself can give you any. But I will say this. Ask the correct questions first, and they will come.'

Without further discussion Lister gave a stiff nod, then turned towards the operating table and back to his body, merging into it from behind - one shadow joining the other. Westman merely faded away, there one moment, gone the next.

'Who is that bloke, Dave?' Alf asked, as he watched Lister put the final few sutures in place.

Gray told him.

'The gargle man?'

'What?'

'Y'know,' Alf hummed a tune, 'Listerine, keeps yer mouth clean.'

'Don't know, Alf. It was probably just named after him because it's antiseptic.'

'Do yer think he's been givin' you a load of mouthwash?'

'No, Alf, I don't. They're both honourable men, and your mother said spirits wouldn't harm me, so I imagine that means they always tell the truth.'

'Suppose you're right,' Alf said, as they both experienced the now familiar modulation in the quality of light, and a rush to the chest.

6

A muddy expanse of bare earth which had once been lush green wood stretched to the horizon in every direction. Like monstrous spent matches planted in the ground by a giant's hand, charred and twisted tree trunks littered the scene, their denuded tops splintered and torn as if harvested with a huge blunt scythe. Here and there flat stretches of silver-white betrayed scores of small ponds, each and every water-filled depression a deep shellhole. Everything was a sepia monochrome, from the foreboding rainclouds above to the dark glistening mud underfoot, and for a moment Gray thought he'd lost his colour vision, until the incongruous candystripes of Alf's pyjamas proved him wrong.

'Where are we ?'

'Buggered if I know, Dave. Looks like a battlefield.'

As the words left Alf's lips a whistling mortar shell landed thirty yards away, cleaving the soil and spewing brown mud and water. Gray ducked to his knees instinctively, but Alf stood his ground as the compression blast and vapour passed harmlessly through them both.

'Still ain't got the 'ang of this have you?' Alf looked down at the crouching figure of his companion, who carefully rose to his feet, noting the unexpected absence of dirt on his clothes. 'Nothing's going to hurt yer, Dave. Not while I'm around.'

As the smoke and smell of cordite wafted away downwind, a distant wailing caused them both to turn and concentrate on the noise.

'What do you reckon, Alf?' Gray said after a few seconds.

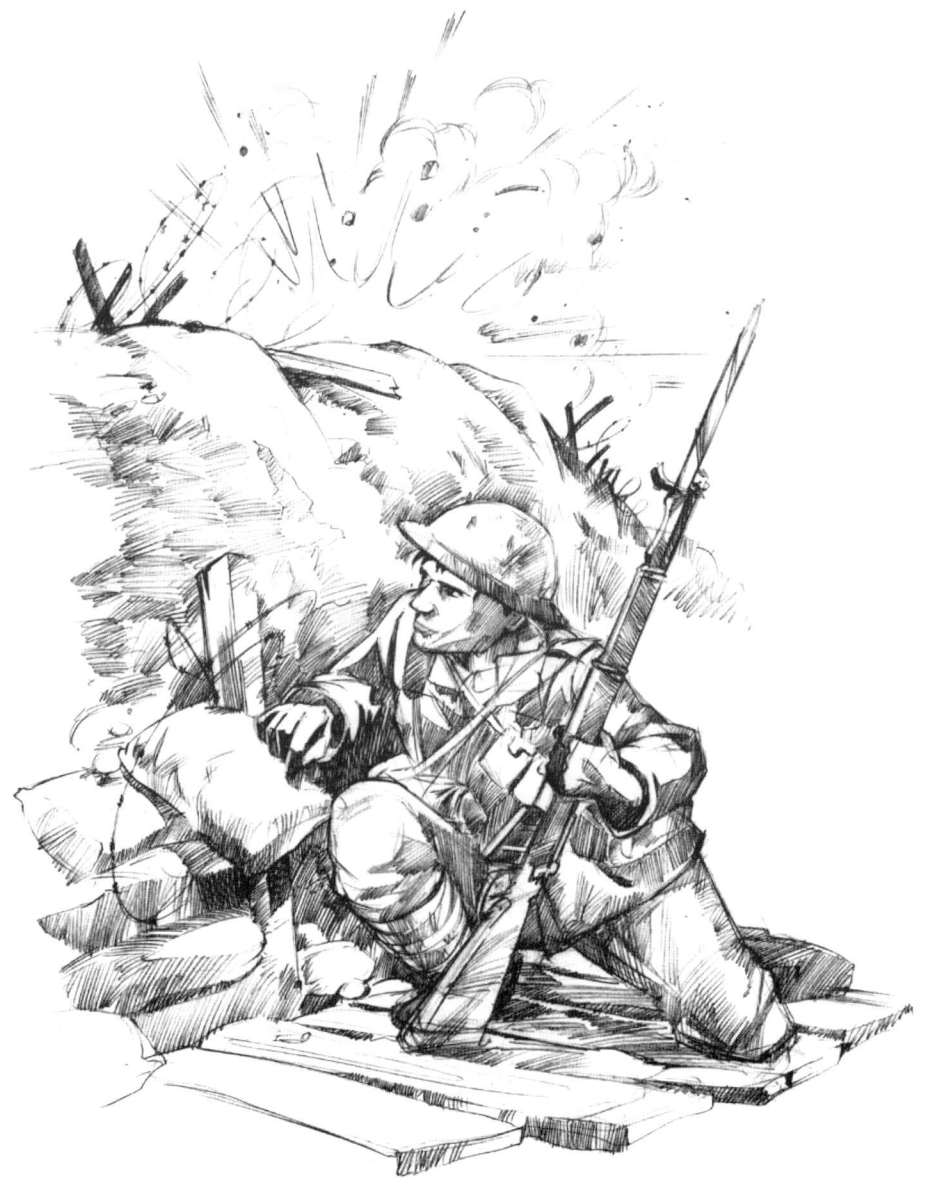

Chapter 6 **71**

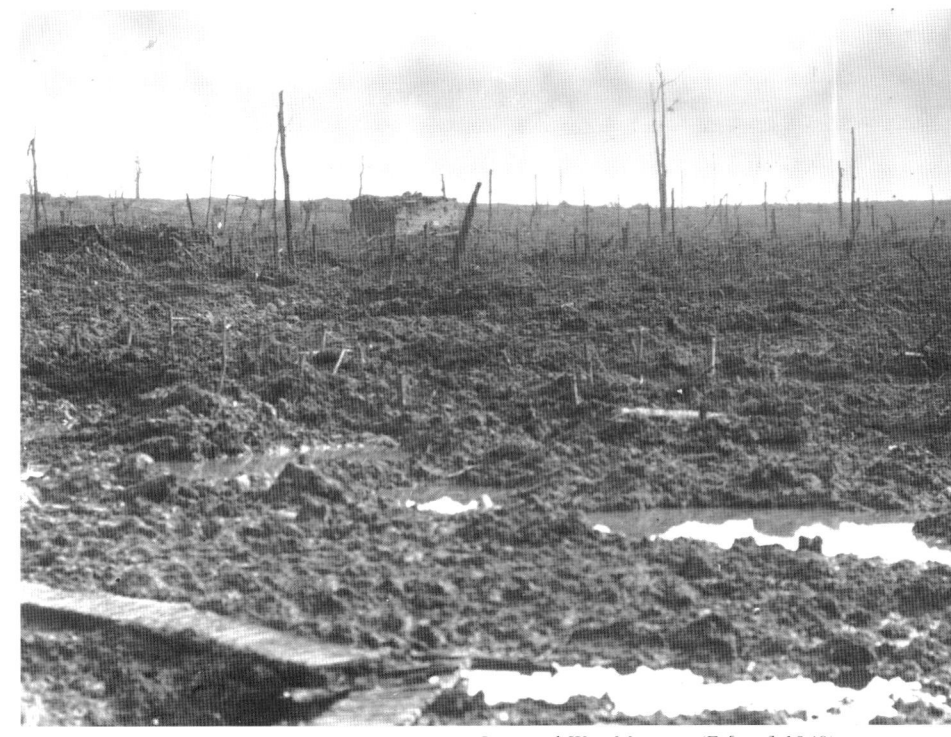

Imperial War Museum (E [aus] 1049)

'Go see who's hurting?'

Gray nodded suspiciously, wary of what further emotional turmoil his fate held, and led the way.

They found him in a deep scoop of ground, on his knees in the glutinous mire with several feet of frothy intestine floating on the wet mud lapping at his thighs. A shard of red-hot mortar steel had sliced through his midriff like a sabre cut. Wide-eyed in disbelief, and with the screaming now a subdued primaeval whimpering, his shaking hands tried to gather up and push the pink squirming coils of gut back into the ragged hole in his bleeding belly. But every frantic movement caused more loops to slither out into the mud. The uniform and telescopic rifle at his side told he was a British Corporal and a sniper, and the soft down and acne on his cheeks put him at no more than nineteen.

'Poor sod,' Alf announced with a kind-hearted sigh. 'I suppose this must be Flanders or suchlike. The *Great* War,' he snorted with disdain. 'This lad,' nodding down at the mewling soldier, 'is a sniper. They get in position before sunrise and sneak back to their own lines after nightfall. Someone must have spotted him in his nest and got lucky with the mortar.'

From their vantage point on the raised ridge of the shellhole, Gray surveyed the hellish scene. Nothing stirred. 'Isn't anyone going to come and get him?'

'Not until after dark, Dave. That's when the orderlies and stretcher bearers do their rounds. If anyone shows their head before then they'll get it blown off.'

Down in the pit the young soldier wrestled with his guts, but gave up the impossible task of pushing them all back into his abdomen. Instead, he tore open the rent in his tunic further, and stuffed the writhing loops inside his shirt until they lay contained and controlled against the bare skin of his belly. Satisfied with the result, with one hand he clasped the tunic shut, instinctively shouldered his rifle with the other, and then clambered through the slime toward the rim of the hole.

'Stay where you are, lad, wait until dark,' Alf urged, but he was talking to himself. 'He's going to try and run for it,' Alf explained to Gray. 'But he won't stand a snowball's chance.'

Gray looked up at the murky clouds. The light was fading. 'It'll be dark soon, why doesn't he just stay put?'

Alf watched the soldier risk a quick bob of his head above the skyline in order to get his bearings. 'He's decided that since he's going to die, he'd rather do it in the company of his mates in the trenches, and not all alone in this stinking hole.'

A crack of rifle shot sounded out from somewhere, and a bullet zizzed through the empty space just vacated by the soldier's steel helmet. 'He won't get two yards,' Gray said. 'Can't we help him?'

'How?'

'I don't know, Alf! But we can't just stand by and watch him die, can we?'

'If it's who I think it is, he doesn't die.'

'What's that supposed to mean. Who do you think he is?'

Alf smiled at Gray's bemused expression. 'He's me pa. That's why I know so much about it.'

The young sniper eventually decided it would be safer to wait for the sun to set, so he settled with his back resting against the side of the shellhole, head well down, and concentrated on gathering his strength while the dull ache in his belly slowly transformed into a blazing furnace. Alf and Gray waited with him.

It was a famous story in the Angel family, and Alf recounted it to pass away the time: how his father was a crack shot who was promoted to Corporal and overcame all odds after being hit by a mortar fragment. 'So you see,' Alf finished the tale, which with embellishments had lasted an hour or more. 'He has to live otherwise I wouldn't be here would I? 'Cos him and ma didn't meet until after he was shipped back to England. Clever ain't it? I remember seeing the scars on his stomach when I was a kid, and the medal he got.'

The soldier on the ground between them began to stir in the darkness and struggle to his feet. He was cold, stiff, and faint through blood loss and the early stages of peritonitis. With stifled gasps of pain he clambered to the rim and stepped over it into the night.

'Looks like it's time to move, Dave,' Alf announced cheerfully. 'I reckon we're supposed to follow him, eh?'

Gray regarded the soldier with a professional eye. 'He's a brave tough lad, Alf, but if he doesn't get help soon he will definitely die.'

'Trust me.' Alf winked and moved off. Gray followed behind.

The allied trench lay less than twenty yards away across no-man's land, but for young Corporal Angel it might as well have been twenty miles of slipping, sliding, tripping, tumbling, blindfolded torment. One fall caused him to cry out so loudly a yellow sodium flare exploded high overhead and floated prettily beneath its small parachute for a minute or more. The corporal had the presence of mind to lay still where he fell; a small wave of inconspicuous mud in a frozen sea of the stuff. Alf and Gray stood guard as the flare descended.

Alf began to laugh.

'What's the matter?' Gray asked, looking around for the source of such hilarity, and noting in passing that neither his or Alf's seemingly solid form cast a shadow in the jaundiced artificial light.

'I remember this bit. The flare. He told me about it when I was knee high!' Alf looked up at the dazzling orb and watched it float downwind, illuminating the base of the low clouds.

'Who did?'

'He did,' Alf said, indicating the man-sized blob at his feet. 'Me pa. He's goin' ter make it Dave, don't you see? He lived to tell me this tale when I were a lad!'

Gray shook his head in amazement. With the flare gone, the soldier began crawling on his knees. Curiously, though it was pitch-dark, Gray could see everything in perfect detail. The man - that is, Alf's father, though Gray was still far from convinced - and the very ground he crawled painfully over, seemed to glow with a faint luminescence he'd never noticed before. Too much artificial light, he supposed. He looked at his own hands and body, and saw a faint glow there too. Then he looked over at Alf.

Delightful, guileless, ludicrous Alf, strolling across a World War One battlefield in the middle of the night wearing hospital pyjamas, and carefully watching over his own father with a proud smile on his whiskered benign face. Alf had the glow too, it was all over him, but brighter than his own, and somehow Gray knew at once it was the pure light of life.

'Leyton Orient', the soldier whispered his password into the darkness, then grunted in pain.

Soft mutterings escaped from the slit trench not two yards away. 'Over 'ere mate,' came a muted reply.

Gray and Alf followed Corporal Angel until a volley of helping hands plucked him headlong into the trench, and were rewarded with screams of agony, followed by gasps of horror.

Chapter 6   **75**

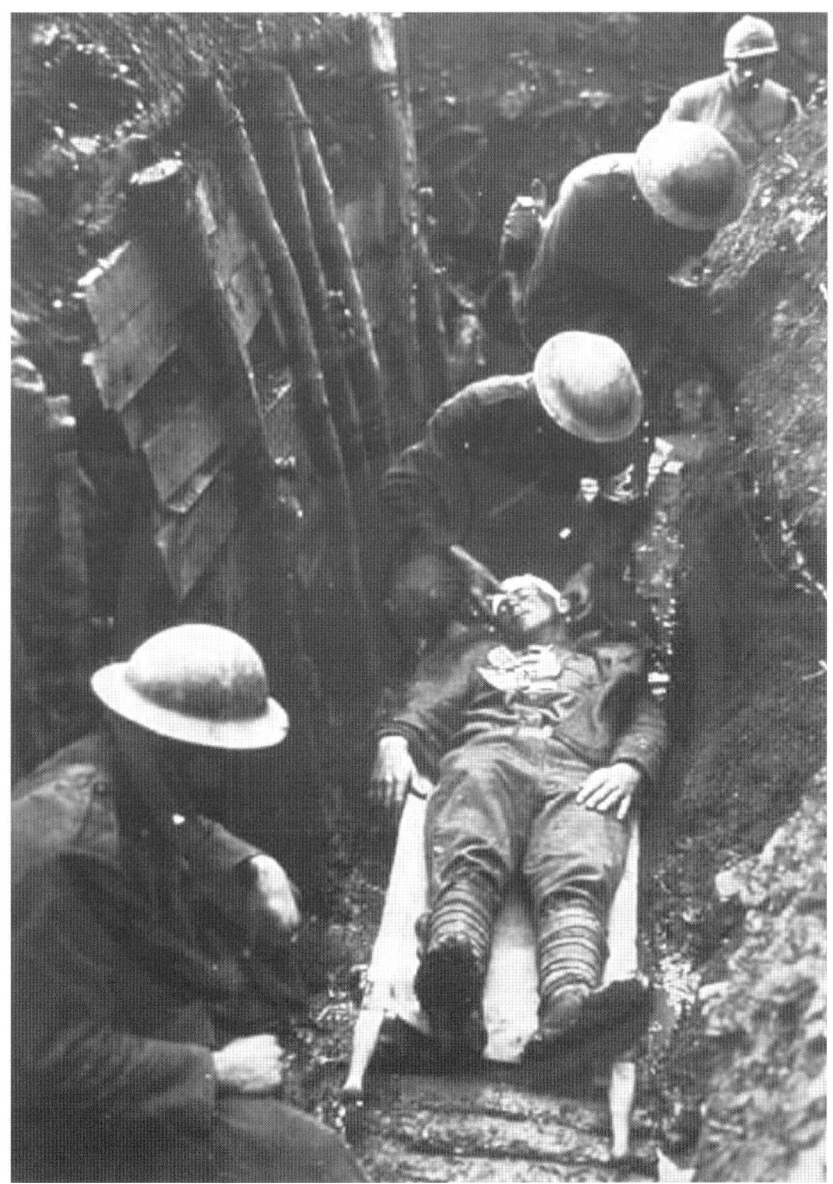

The National Library of Medicine (US)

It took three hours to transport the corporal back through the lines. The orderlies and stretcher crew at the advanced dressing post knew he was "a goner" as soon as they saw "the guts 'angin outer 'is belly". So they took their time carrying him through the trenches, dimly lit here and there with shaded candles, and made sure he had a cigarette and plenty of morphine before loading him onto the horse-drawn ambulance for the torturing ride to the Casualty Clearing Station.

Five miles behind the front line and spread over three acres, the CCS was a regimented collection of khaki marquees and Nissen huts erected around the central hub of a commandeered farmhouse with a deep well and a plentiful supply of fresh water. Although capable of relatively swift mobility, the station had not moved in eighteen months: such was the fluidity of trench warfare.

On arrival the ambulance queued in the dark farmyard with a dozen others until, having reached the front of the line, it was then able to spew its load of walking wounded and stretcher cases into the large barn for preliminary assessment, or triage.

Inside, the barn was well lit with oil lamps hanging from the rafters, and the casualties were either stretchered out in neat rows over the centre of the earthen floor, or else sat untidily around the sides with their backs to the wooden walls. A youthful major and his more elderly sergeant strolled through the mayhem of groaning broken men. Both men wore grubby blood-spattered greatcoats and balaclavas, though the officer sported soft leather riding boots instead of ankle boots and puttees. The major cast a hasty glance at the corporal's shredded contaminated bowel and immediately triaged his semi-conscious body to the moribund tent, to die there alongside the scores of other stinking head, chest and belly wounds. The sergeant scribbled "M" in red stickpaint on the patient's forehead and moved on with a shake of his head: *they always arrive at night, the living dead always arrive at night.*

Gray and Alf, who had hitched a covert lift in the ambulance, looked on aghast as the major moved down the line to the next stretcher case, a shattered femur, and with a flick of his head indicated the pre-op tent. The sergeant barked an order and two stretcher bearers hurriedly obliged.

'What's happening, Dave?' Alf was frantic.

'They're selecting the men who can be saved, Alf. I'm afraid your dad's not one of them.' Gray turned away from Alf's anxious face, ashamed of the truth.

'That can't be!' he cried. 'He lives, Dave. I told you he lives!'

'Perhaps you're wrong, Alf.' Gray crouched at the corporal's side to avoid his friend's glare. 'Perhaps this isn't your father. Just some other poor sod who never lived long enough to fall in love and have children.'

Alf stuck a beefy hand in Gray's armpit and pulled him to his feet. 'It's him, I'm telling you. Now do something! Help him!'

'How, Alf?' Gray voiced his own mounting ire. Being surrounded by injuries and wounds he had the skill and knowledge to treat and cure, yet having to witness such primitive ignorance, was getting at him. 'What the bloody hell can I do? I can't even touch them. Look!' By way of demonstration he passed his palm through the bandaged head of a nearby mustard gas victim. 'Have you got any idea how difficult all this is for me? All these men dying needlessly. I need to get my hands on them but I can't!'

'I think I know a way,' Alf said calmly.

'Oh yeah. How?'

'Get into him.' Alf pointed at the major, now several yards away, tying a ligature with his bare hands onto a spurting artery in a neck wound. 'Remember that copper you walked into? Well walk into the doc over there and talk to him. Tell him what to do and how to do it.'

Gray's eyebrows did a somersault. 'Is that possible?'

'Dunno, Dave. But we've got to try something, because if he dies now,' Alf nodded down at his father, then tapped his own chest, 'I reckon I won't be hanging around with you for much longer!'

Gray gulped hard as the reasoning behind Alf's words sank in. Then he turned and walked slowly down the row of stretchers.

Major Gordon Gordon-Taylor wiped his bloody hands on the coarse fibres of his coat and observed his handiwork. He'd just tied off the common carotid artery of the soldier lying in front of him. Now, with half the brain deprived of blood, would the man become paralysed down one side? *No*, the answer leapt into his mind, *he's young, he'll have a good collateral circulation.* As he watched, the soldier continued struggling against the hands of the orderlies holding him down. Both legs were still kicking. *Good.*

Gordon-Taylor rose from his knees to survey the remaining carnage. A tall lean aesthetic man with aquiline features, the scene offended his sensibilities. Filthy wounds everywhere, broken bones and macerated flesh mixed with blood and mud, most of which the nurses and junior officers could handle adequately; simple clean and cut out the dead meat work. It seemed to him his own job had degenerated to choosing between those who were hopeless cases and those who had a chance. *Shouldn't you be trying harder? How else will things get better? Who says gut wounds are necessarily lethal? Clean and debride is the rule, why should bowel be different?* His gaze ranged back down the line to the corporal. *Why not try? What's there to lose? He'll die anyway.*

'Sergeant, I've changed my mind about that man with the belly wound. Move him to the theatre tent now, I'll do it myself. And take some blood to match off one of the healthier men in the fracture ward. Tell whoever volunteers I'll sign a chit for two weeks extra leave.'

'Sir?'

'Just do it man, and find someone to take over from me here. It's time we made a difference!'

Alf looked on with a barely perceptible smile. It was all going to work.

oooooooooooooooooooooooooooooooooo

In the theatre marquee, generator-driven electric lamps were strung like bunting across the low canvas roof, with concentrations of bulbs above each of the ten operating trolleys. Thick white-washed wooden boards lining the floor and sidewalls served to lend some permanency and sturdiness to the structure, but also reflected light and the new paradigm of aseptic surgery. The

Chapter 6   **79**

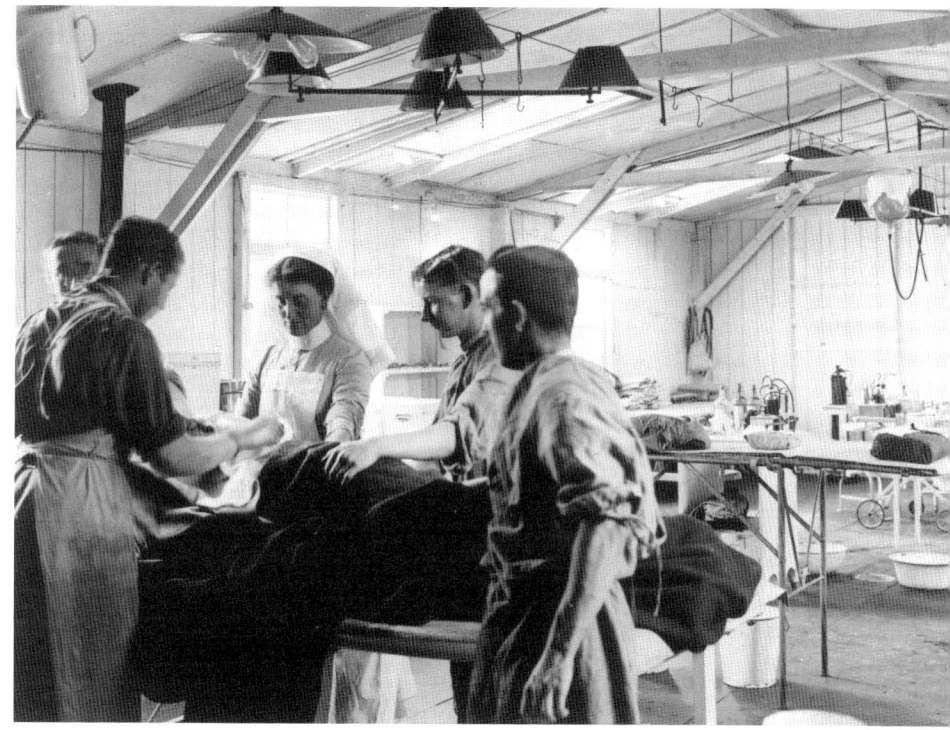

Imperial War Museum (CO 382)

air, warm and moist from steamers used to sterilize instruments and drapes, was redolent with the whiff of soap and spirit, and hand-basins full of boiled water were everywhere.

At every table a surgeon and assistant laboured, each in a sterile white smock from neck to knees, with sleeves rolled up above scrubbed-clean forearms and hands - no gloves, nor headcaps or facemasks. Some patients were awake, the operating site rendered insensitive with spinal cocaine, the original local anaesthetic. Others were asleep, anaesthetised with balanced mixtures of oxygen and ether administered by doctors specializing in the craft.

Circulating around the tent were Queen Alexandra's nurses, emulating Florence Nightingale in full grey skirts, white cotton aprons and elaborate hats bearing a red cross emblem. Fiercely proud of being the only women allowed so close to the front line, the QAs acted as scrub nurses, fetched instruments and ties where required, applied or removed dressings, cleaned unremittingly, and when necessary, prayed.

Above everything else, Alf noted as he nosed around the theatre, was the noise. Against the backround throb of the generator, surgeons were yelling for help, loudly swearing at themselves and their assistants, or changing tables and gently encouraging each other's efforts. Nurses clattered over the floor pushing metal trolleys full of surgical instruments and shouting orders at each other, or in honeyed female tones soothed anxious young men as they witnessed their own limbs being amputated. The clamour was mixed and raucous, but, Alf registered, the screams of steel cutting into sensate flesh were absent.

His father's operation was on-going, but Alf was unconcerned. Indeed he was supremely confident, because with Dave on the job, together with the fact that he - that is, Alf himself - still existed, a successful outcome was assured. And as a bonus, whether he realised it or not, young Dave was discovering his compassion again.

Meanwhile, Gordon-Taylor was sweating nervously in unchartered territory, unsure his skills were up to the challenge. Upon opening the abdomen he discovered the corporal's peritoneal cavity full of foul green intestinal fluid, with lengths of small bowel either holed like a colander or black with gangrene, and knew immediately he'd made a mistake. The received wisdom was correct; the man was doomed. *Come on! You're here now and at least the colon's intact. Resect the bowel and wash out the peritoneum. Clean and debride must work here as well. Why shouldn't it?*

'You tickety-boo, Gordon?' the anaesthetist enquired brightly in clipped public school speak, aware his friend was ignoring the rule book and risking both his reputation and career. 'Bit of a mess inside, what?'

'This might take some time, George. Bear with me would you?' *Tell him to give the blood now, and fluids. Tell him to treat the shock.* 'What about giving that blood now, eh? In case I spill any.'

'Anything for Gee Squared Tee old chap,' he said, using his friend's nickname. 'Oh and by the way, if anyone can do this, old man, you can. I'm with you all the way.'

From his unique vantage point, Gray watched Gordon-Taylor at work, felt the blood on his bare hands, sensed his trepidation, admired his skill and speed. *Don't fret, it's easy, you've got good hands. Cut out the devitalised bowel, perform an end-to-end anastomosis with catgut, then wash everything scrupulously clean with saline. Infection is the enemy, so leave the belly open and do a secondary suture in a few days when you're sure it's healthy. Just like you do with compound fractures. Back to first principles. It will work, you know it will.*

For Gordon-Taylor, like many surgeons, talking or thinking to himself when operating was second nature; a nerve-calming mantra employed particularly - especially - when up excrement creek without a paddle and with the cold slimy reptile of fear caressing his spine. But that night, unconsciously advancing the accepted boundaries of surgical science in a field of war-torn Europe, the voice in his head didn't seem entirely his own. The confident and assuring tone was alien to his usual self-effacing, self-doubting nature. Yet the reasoning made obvious sense. So he ascribed his revelation to necessity being the mother of invention, shrugged his shoulders, and simply got on with it.

'Well?' Alf asked. They were standing behind the anaesthetist, watching Gordon-Taylor dressing the open wound.

'He'll live, Alf,' Gray said inattentively, recalling the weird experience he'd undergone. Of all the events so far, it was the most bizarre.

By trial and error he had eventually manoeuvred himself through the red haze until he could see through Gordon-Taylor's eyes, and once in position, realised with astonishment he had access to all the other senses, including the man's thoughts and emotions. It was like pulling on an all-feeling skin-tight suit, but not in a parasitic way; more a symbiotic blend of minds with the "host" unaware of a second guiding personality. Gray was sure of it because he had sensed no feelings of disquiet or fear, just the usual uneasiness of tackling a new and difficult procedure. For a short time their consciousness was one and the same, and he'd acted normally, doing the surgery and imparting his experience wrought through the serendipity of having trained in a more enlightened age. But his own enlightenment came from the reported experiences and teaching of surgeons like Gordon-Taylor. So which came first? The tautology was so mind-bending he eventually gave up on it.

Then he remembered Westman's description of dead medics acting as muses to live counterparts, and understood he had just performed the same function. Yet if he could do it so easily without being discovered, had Gray himself been similarly influenced during his career? And if so, when, how, and by whom?

7

Life just wasn't worth living anymore. Forty-six years old, going through a divorce, with his wife taking him to the cleaners, the business going belly-up, the tax man after him for certain "discrepancies" in the accounts, and now, to top it all, his new woman - the one who'd begged him to walk away from his marriage and children - had told him their relationship was over. Part of the attraction she said, had been his wealth, but the way things were panning out he was turning into a poor, sad old man, with the emphasis on poor. And she wasn't prepared to put up with it, or help out.

That had been an hour ago, at the end of their romantic candle-lit dinner in the restaurant of the expensive hotel where he'd booked the honeymoon suite for the night using a credit card. Selfish bitch! Typical of her to wait until the end of the meal, and the wine, and the liqueurs. To wait until he'd paid the bill.

He saw the lorry, saw it clearly, halted at the road junction a hundred yards ahead, its rear lights shining brightly in the darkness. His right foot automatically moved to the brake pedal, then hovered over it as a notion suddenly flashed through his mind. Did he really want to wake up alone in the single bed of that grubby little rented flat? No, he decided. Why not end it all then; tonight? Why not now? It would be an accident wouldn't it? Not suicide from a brandy and barbiturate overdose. The life insurance would have to cough up; debts cleared, mortgage paid off, the kids' education ensured. All his troubles would be over, painlessly and permanently. His foot eased back to the throttle, and pressed hard.

Young Gray slouched in one of the dozen ancient armchairs in the doctors' mess, eyelids half closed, his white coat crumpled and grubby. Saturday night soccer was on the TV, but he watched it alone. His houseman was a girl with no interest in Liverpool versus Arsenal, so she'd foolishly gone to bed. The on-call medical team must be busy, he reasoned, and he knew the gynaecologists and anaesthetists were occupied with an emergency Caesarian section. No other medics were resident in the hospital during weekends. Hence his lonely vigil.

It would come soon. He knew it. Every Saturday night was the same. Pubs shut at eleven, car crashes by half-past, urgent bleeper call to casualty by twelve. He hated it. Hated the unnecessary death and mutilation, the ruination of so many lives, the sheer bloody stupidity. *Bleep, bleep, bleep.*

The resuscitation room was the usual hive of casualty officers, nurses and radiographers. Unconscious on the trolley lay a middle-aged man with half his face hanging off, and an endotracheal tube sticking out of the bloodied mess where his mouth and lips should have been. They were cutting off the soiled expensive suit and sticking IV lines into his arms when he arrived.

'Bit odd this one, Dave,' the casualty registrar said. 'Not the usual kid in a clapped out Cortina. Ran his Mercedes into the back of a lorry. Not wearing a belt. Went through the windscreen.'

'Drunk?' Gray scanned his eyes over the exposed body; blood, dirt and shattered safety glass everywhere.

'Probably. Not that it matters much. So far, working from the bottom up we've got a right femur, compound left tib and fib, blood from his dick so he's probably fractured his pelvis, belly's blowing up, possible left pneumothorax, the face of course, fractured jaw and maxilla there, and I don't know about his head yet, but the pupils are normal. So, over to you.' He smiled maliciously, 'You weren't expecting any sleep tonight, were you?'

'Up yours,' Gray said in less than good humour, acknowledging the fact that the casualty boys worked a shift system, whereas a resident's job entailed twenty-four hour cover for the whole weekend, Friday through to Monday. By eight in the morning his tormentor would be comfortably asleep in bed, whereas Gray himself would probably be in theatre with this same patient, still have a full day and night of emergency work ahead of him, and then a normal Monday of elective surgery and clinics.

He snapped out orders, first to the rather attractive radiographer who he knew to be more decorative than functional: 'Get him x-rayed from head to foot, and I want a good neck film with C7 and T1 on it, no half-hearted crap or you'll have to do it again.' Then to the nursing sister, an experienced senior woman he trusted: 'June, get my houseman out of her bed and get hold of one of the anaesthetists; last time I heard they were in maternity doing a section. We need them here, now!' Finally, the casualty registrar again: 'Trevor, do me a favour. Get a central line in and fill him up with O-neg until the cross-matched blood's ready. Keep him out of shock for me until the others arrive. While you're doing that I'm going to make a few calls.'

Finding an empty office with a phone, Gray shut the door, sat down with a weary hopelessness, lit a cigarette, and took a few moments to marshal his thoughts into some sort of game plan. He had yet to examine the man properly, not that it mattered much; before long he'd be on an operating table with his belly open. What horrors, Gray wondered, would that Pandora's box hold? And could he deal with them? Spleen, yes. Guts, yes. Kidneys, probably. Liver and pancreas...? Oh well, there was always the boss to call in from home. The broken legs were no problem; clean, debride, fix. From the sound of things a fractured pelvis had disrupted the urethra, but he'd sort that out on the table. The only insurmountable problem was the mashed face. That was a job for specialists; the max-fax boys. Gray picked up the phone and spoke to the hospital switchboard: 'Put me through to whichever maxillo-facial consultant's on call, and then I need to speak to theatres.'

ooooooooooooooooooooooooooooooooo

'Where are we now?' Alf's tone betrayed a certain irritation with all the comings and goings. He wasn't tired physically (that would be an oxymoron), but dealing with Dave's mixed emotions and more latterly his own was mentally draining, and he could do with a rest from it. After all, he didn't know what his own future held, apart from the fact he was going to die, or rather his body was going to die. From a heart attack. On Friday. Whenever that was. Or was going to be. What happens then? An eternity of errands like this? What was it his mother had called him - a companion and guide? Well, he decided, if this is what dying is like, you can stuff it.

'Seems there's no rest for the wicked, Alf,' Gray mumbled, taking in the scene and inadvertently reflecting his partner's mood.

It was a modern operating theatre with two teams working on the same patient. A surgeon, his junior, and a scrub nurse were gathered around the head end, a similar crew around the abdomen. The wall mounted twenty-four hour clock showed 01:49. Gray immediately recognised the setting, and intuitively understood he was there as a consequence of his own thoughts. For this was the night he grew up. The operation which matured David Gray into a fully competent surgeon.

The max-fax consultant at the top end, by virtue of age, rank and status, was the senior man. Young Gray, with his boyish features and fashionably long hair poking out beneath the blue theatre cap, felt very much his junior. Nevertheless, the two conferred as equals, which up to a point they were, since the max-fax man could offer no substantial help or advice to his junior general surgical colleague. Gray would have to deal with whatever he found in the distended bloated abdomen on his own, but his every move could, and no doubt would, be monitored for competence, and his performance eventually relayed back to his own boss. Just one more thing to worry about. Another turn on the pressure screw. Marvellous! Sweat stuck the theatre greens to his back.

They both agreed a tracheostomy was needed - with most of the facial bones and jaw shattered, a secure airway was the first priority - and young Gray waited patiently with gloved hands clamped to his chest as the maxillo-facial specialist quickly dissected down to the trachea and supervised the withdrawal of the endotracheal tube. The patient himself was already anaesthetised and well out of the fray. The two inch slash beneath the Adam's

Chapter 7

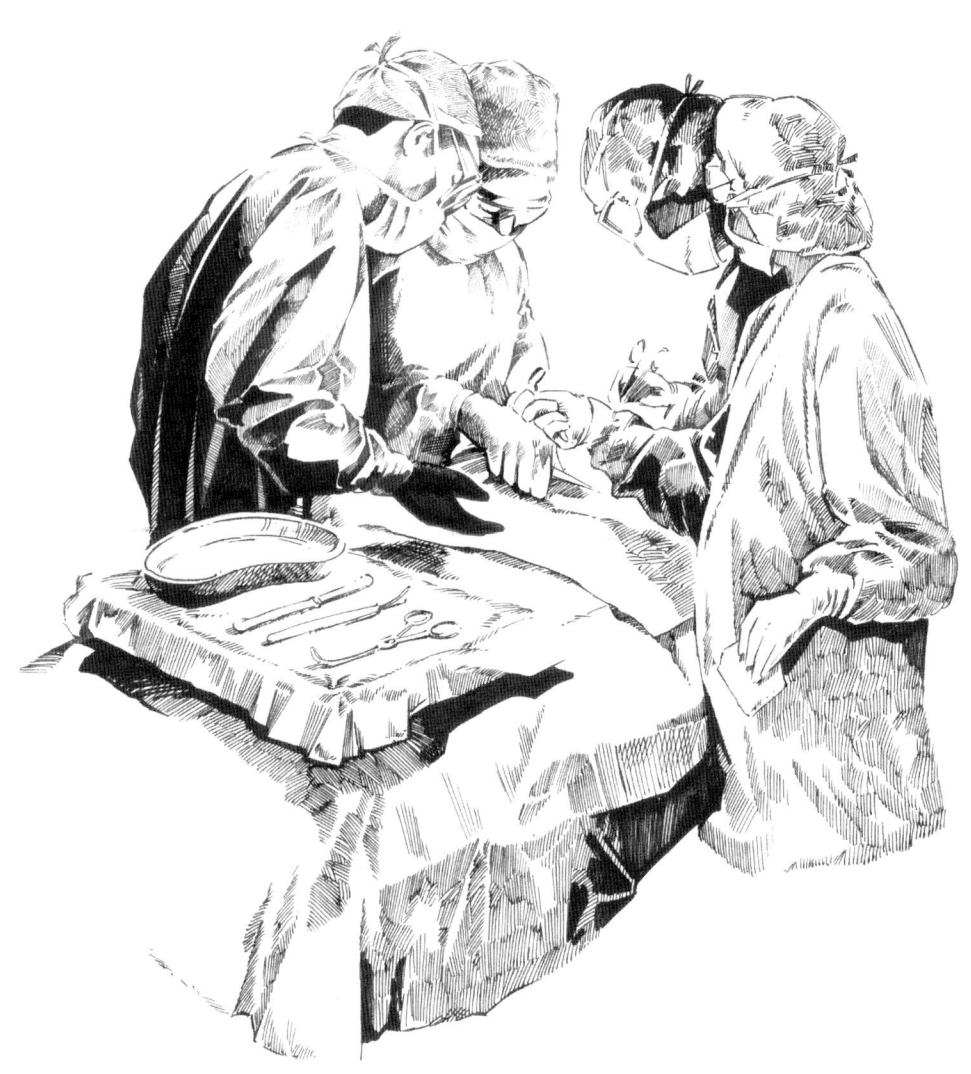

apple readily accepted the tracheostomy tube, and the gasman swiftly connected his pipes to it before checking the dials and flow-meters with satisfaction. 'Okay, I'm happy. Now, let's get on with it folks, this guy's clapped out and still hosing from somewhere.' His eyes, along with everyone else's, went to the melon-ripe belly and then fixed on Gray. They all knew it was down to him.

In the background Gray senior and Alf leaned against one of the cream-coloured walls. Alf noted with mild amusement that his new friend hadn't fallen through it, though he thought it best not to point it out.

'Well, Dave, are you gonna tell me what's going on? I can see that's a young you over there, even with the mask, but yer a bit older than before. Looks like yer in charge.'

Gray turned his gaze to Alf. 'I was a junior registrar, a few months after passing all my exams, about six or seven years off a consultant job, and thought I was the bee's knees. The patient was from a car crash and needed a specialist to screw his face and wire his jaw together. I had to deal with the rest. It was a huge operation, and I was shit scared I wouldn't be able to hack it.'

Alf nodded towards the operating table. 'You look confident enough.'

'All bluff, Alf. I was still wet behind the ears. Watch what happens.'

Young Gray asked the scrub nurse for a knife and she passed him the scalpel. He hesitated momentarily before drawing it in a straight line from just below the sternal bone to the pubis, skirting the umbilicus as he passed it. Under the flying-saucer operating lights suspended from the ceiling, the skin reflected shiny cream, and yielded like tissue paper to the razor-sharp blade, splitting to reveal the yellow layer of fat beneath. Within seconds, bleeding capillaries spotted the glowing fat with droplets of scarlet, the blood coalescing like sweat and running through the depths of the wound. He cut again, through muscle and tendon until, tense and as purple as a ripe plumb, the thin layer of peritoneum bulged with the blood contained within.

Chapter 7

'Be ready with the sucker,' he instructed the houseman, her drowsy eyes unaware of the depth of his panic. Jesus, what the hell is bleeding so much?

Incising the peritoneum, thin red blood gushed into his face, spread over the green drapes and ran down the front of his surgeon's gown. He blinked to clear his vision.

'SUCK!'

Shocked into action from her slumbering lassitude, the houseman plunged the six-inch chrome tube into the crimson void as Gray hauled out lengths of salmon-pink bowel. Then he inserted his right hand and arm into the wound, displacing a spectacular cascade of even more blood, and felt high up on the left side, under the diaphragm. As he suspected, the spleen was in tatters, its normal firm smooth surface a soft pulp of macerated tissue beneath his fingertips. Shit!

'Retract, hold it there, let's get some light in this corner, suck!' He barked out instructions, and hoped no-one noticed the fine tremor of his hands.

Leaning on the wall still, transfixed by the surgery and the blood, Alf and Gray failed to notice they had gained another companion. Until he spoke.

'Excuse me, I wonder if either of you can help me?'

The two friends turned together, startled.

The man stood cool and nonchalant, jacket slung over one shoulder, collar and tie loosened at the neck of his tailored white shirt, one hand in the pocket of his trousers. He oozed wealth and confidence, from his perfect coiffure of black hair, all the way down to his hand-made shoes. The always-in-control business executive continued, 'Everyone else seems to belong here,' gesturing to the theatre staff in greens, 'but you two clearly don't, so I assume you're in the same predicament as me.'

Alf spoke first, his eyebrows beetled into a suspicious frown, 'That all depends, dunnit?'

'On what?'

'On what "prerdikerment" yer in.'

The man cleared his throat awkwardly. 'Well, the fact is, I expected to be dead, but it appears I'm not.'

As the businessman spoke, the space and light to one side of him appeared to shimmer and grow dense, until the shape and outline of a second human form was unmistakeable. 'Not another one!' Gray groaned. 'This is turning into a damned convention.'

'It's a pleasure to see you as well,' Gerry Westman announced with a broad grin.

Alf was still in a challenging mood. 'I thought we'd already said our goodbye's, Gerry. Why are you still followin' us?'

'It's probably more the other way around, Alf,' he said with a chuckle. 'Anyway, there's no such thing as goodbye, is there? Only *au revoir*. Think about it. Now listen up chaps, I'd love to have a long chat but right now I've work to do.' Westman turned, strode confidently towards the operating table, and melted into the back of young Gray.

Almost immediately the immature surgeon moved with more confidence, his hands working with a surprising rapidity and sureness, the nervous tremor gone. He could do it! It was easy! Training, knowledge and skill all coming together at once. The shattered spleen was soon out, the gushing pedicle tied off, and the catastrophic haemorrhage stemmed. What next? The torn gut first, then repair the bladder, railroad a catheter through the urethra, remember to check the pancreas, make a start on the fractures...

'Blood pressure's recovering,' the anaesthetist proclaimed to the assembly.

Gray turned to the dumbfounded businessman, anxious to give a kindly reassuring word. But the man was already disappearing, transformed into a cloud of translucent mist and sparkling silver points of light which spiralled head first into his own eviscerated body, lying broken and mutilated on the table.

'He survived, Alf,' Gray explained. 'Walked out of hospital three months later, back to his wife and kids. I remember him telling me he'd been a bit of a prat before the crash. Turned out it was a suicide attempt. His wife eventually showed up on the ward, said she loved him and wanted him back to look after him. It was all very emotional and tearful. I didn't know Westman was helping me with the operation though. I certainly didn't feel him at the time. Don't remember feeling anything really, except being scared out of my wits. We got him off the table at about seven in the morning. I was completely knackered, but after that I knew I could cope with anything. Never got frightened again.'

Alf appeared sheepish, scratched the stubble on his chin, and hitched his pyjama pants up. 'Well, it seems I've misjudged Gerry and owe him an apology. Suppose there's no time like the present.' He shuffled over to the operating table and pressed his face gently into the back of young Gray's head, then withdrew it almost at once and came back. 'The bugger's already left! There's only you in there.'

'Au revoir!' David smiled gently.

'Yeah, what was that all about?' Alf said.

'It means, until we meet again. No such thing as goodbye. I suppose all of us eventually meet again. Like you and your family, Alf.'

'Oh yeah!' The light of understanding brightened his crinkled features. 'I'm bein' a bit thick I suppose.'

'Far from it, Alf. You just said something fundamentally important.'

'Me?'

'Yes. You said there's no time like the present.'

'It's just a saying, ain't it?'

'Not from our perspective, Alf. Time doesn't seem to have any meaning does it? Past or present, it's all the same. And Gerry Westman's flitting about all over the place. He doesn't die for years yet, but we've both just seen him clear as day. His body right now is still alive somewhere, yet a few minutes ago his spirit was helping me over there.' Gray nodded towards his younger self standing at the operating table. 'So how does it all work, eh?'

'Perhaps he was dreaming,' Alf said uncertainly.

'Who?'

'Gerry. If he's still alive now, perhaps he's safely tucked up in bed and dreaming he's helping you. Don't you ever get dreams about work? I used to have 'em all the time, specially after I retired. Really vivid ones like I was really there, diggin' 'oles and laying bricks with all these guys who knew my name and treated me like an old mate. The funny thing was I didn't know who they were, but that didn't matter see, 'cos I was enjoying myself and seemed to fit in somehow. Felt as if I belonged.' Alf chortled to himself at the memory. 'Some mornings I'd worked so hard in me sleep, I'd wake up with a stiff back an' sore 'ands. Now if your mate Gerry just 'appened to be up and about like, y'know, us...'

Listening to Alf's rambling notion, Gray's imagination slipped into overdrive. Yes, he had experienced similar dreams. Who hasn't? Vaguely familiar people in vaguely familiar surroundings and situations. Got a problem? Sleep on it. It was part of everyday human experience. Was it possible that consciousness, or should that be one's spirit, is capable of wandering off in what we perceive as dreams?

Unseen by anyone except Alf, Gray paced the length and breadth of the operating theatre, muttering and grunting, scratching his head, stopping now and then to pursue a particular line of thought, a new angle; the scientist doing what he knew best, logical enquiry.

'Alf!' He stopped suddenly in front of his friend. 'Where is now? Where exactly is the present? Is it here, back in the trenches with your father, or thirty years from now with me meeting you after my own car crash? We've been doing a fair bit of flitting about ourselves since then haven't we? But everywhere we go seems real enough to me. How about you?'

'Well,' Alf's brow furrowed in thought. 'Yeah,' he concluded. 'S'real enough alright.'

'Not a dream? A figment of imagination?'

'Nah. We've done that bit, when I shook your hand. Remember? It hurt you.' Without warning Gray slapped Alf across the cheek, not hard, but enough to startle. Alf jumped back in surprise, rubbing his face, 'What was that for?'

Chapter 7

'Just checking on something. And paying you back.'
'Very funny!'
'Yes, it is,' said Gray, laughing. 'Come on, Alf, if I'm right we're off somewhere new.'

ooooooooooooooooooooooooooooooooo

They arrived in a small tutorial room complete with whiteboards, flipcharts, an overhead projector, a video screen, and a few dozen plastic chairs. It was the type of small cluttered seminar space found in any organisation anywhere in the world, except Gray knew the room and recognised the scene from the previous week at the hospital - a lunchtime tutorial for the handful of students on his firm and any others who cared to attend. His teaching style, though condemned by the educationalists as old-fashioned chalk and talk - "Sorry, I can't and won't do all that touchy-feely stuff" - was popular, and the hour-long sessions usually attracted equal numbers of junior doctors and students assigned to other consultants. And there he was, in his best suit, standing at the whiteboard in front of a dozen attentive young faces and halfway through his regular "abdominal pain" talk. Like his other lectures, it was honed to perfection after twenty-odd years of repetition, complete with interactive questions, jokes and laughter at specifically allotted points.

It wasn't however, what Gray expected, and it showed in his blank expression.

'Well, it sure is new to me, Dave, but I can see on yer face it ain't very new to you, is it? Alf wearily took a seat at the back of the room. 'That's you in a whistle, ain't it? You look like yer enjoying yerself.' A ripple of laughter came from the audience. 'Teaching, eh? Didn't know you did that as well.'

'We're not supposed to be here, Alf.'

'Oh yeah, where are we supposed to be then?'

Gray had anticipated a look at future medicine and surgery. Things like robotics, gene therapy, drugs to cure cancer and viral infections; yet here he was in his regular tutorial room, listening to himself and knowing which diagram, which joke, even which damned word came next. In exasperation he flung one arm about the room. 'The future, Alf. It's supposed to be the bloody future,' and with a stoop of abject defeat, made to sit in the chair next to his companion, but finally decided not to risk it. 'Alf,' he continued, 'each time I've thought about something, we've ended up somewhere appropriate. We were talking about the past and present, so I made a conscious effort to conjure up the future. But this,' he jerked his chin towards his alter ego, 'this happened only just last week'

Alf's face contorted with disbelief. 'Yer daft sod. What were you expecting, Captain Whatsisname and the Starship Enterprise? How can there be a future when it hasn't 'appened yet!'

For a moment, Gray considered opening a discussion on the metaphysical and quantum conceptualisation of the arrow of time, and whether the future actually existed as an entity in its own right, but the familiar everyday surroundings put paid to any worthwhile debate. 'Sorry, Alf. Perhaps it's your turn to slap me. I was expecting to see how medicine and surgery would look in years to come.'

Alf peered about the room with a pitiful shake of his head before the light of comprehension gleamed in his eyes. 'No wonder!' Then he put out a contemptuous look. 'Ma was right, you do need looking after. And here's me thinking you was an intelligent well-educated man.'

'You know why we're here?'

'I reckon so.' Alf smirked and folded his arms.

'Well?'

'Think about it, Dave. Work it out for yerself.'

'No! You tell me.'

With a slow shake of his head, Alf refused to co-operate. Instead he turned his attention to the lecture, his cracked features transforming into a child-like rapture of concentration.

Perturbed and enraged, Gray began pacing the room like a trapped bear.

'Hey, Dave,' Alf shouted after a while. 'This is good stuff. Even I can understand it. Specially the one about what's brown and buggers old people. Faecal peritonitis!' He giggled with delight.

Across the room, standing at the window with his back turned, Gray shoved his hands deeper into the pockets of his sweat-shirt and stayed silent - it was a very old surgical joke, used because it was both memorable and true. He was studying the consultant's section in the hospital car park fifteen floors below. There, alongside the Mercs, BMWs and Range Rovers, he noted his own Jaguar standing in its usual slot, unbent and undamaged. Sweet Jesus, what was happening to him, and why was he here? The moment needed a nicotine fix, but his pockets were empty - no need for it, he supposed, like the absent Rolex - and in any case, he realised, the craving wasn't there. Strange that, but then again, wasn't everything else?

So what now? He needed guidance. The talk would soon be finished and his smart-suited counterpart would be off to the private clinic to do a list of varicose veins - the memory of the afternoon was still with him, even the faces of the patients. What was he supposed to do then. Wait here forever?

'Alf,' he said softly, his eyes still on the car. 'Please tell me I haven't screwed things up. If there's a reason we're here, what is it?'

'No, Dave, you've not screwed things up. Just think about it more, you're bound to get it eventually.' Alf spoke with equal melancholy, noting the deflated shrug of his friend's shoulders.

Another minute passed before Gray turned sharply from the window. 'Alf, I think I've got it,' he shouted. 'I'm supposed to look inside my own head. That must be why we're here, that's where the answer is.' Gray smiled with satisfaction. 'What do you say?'

'That's a bleedin' barmy idea. The head you've got right now is muddled enough, ain't it? And you want to put all your mixed-up emotions in with his!' Alf indicated the lecturer and shook his head. 'Nah. Sounds like a recipe for disaster to me. Bloody stupid notion.'

Gray ignored the advice. Okay, it was a preposterous idea. Absurd even.

Who or what could he possibly find in there, other than himself? And yet, he reasoned, since the whole situation was equally bizarre, what was there to lose? After all, nothing else seemed to be happening. Perhaps it was time to take things into his own hands, time for some action.

Gently, quietly, he crept to the front of the room, skirting around members of the audience, until he was face-to-face with himself. The old man in the mirror again - but not quite. This was no reflection, no left-right reverse. He was looking into his own face, animate and alive, as others saw him. Gray hesitated, nose to nose with himself.

'Don't do it, Dave.' Gray heard the gruff voice yelling from the back of the room, even as he felt the breath of his own body on his cheeks.

In his own inimitable style, David Gray the man was in full flow, freely bestowing his time and knowledge of abdominal pain with its multiple causes - recognising the discomfort in his own gut as hunger pangs and wondering if he could grab a sandwich before leaving for the private list - when the overwhelming sense of déjà vu hit him. His words faltered momentarily. He'd been here before, exactly here and exactly now. Before. He just knew it. Same faces, same talk, same hunger in his belly, same sunny day with light pouring in through the windows, same clock on the wall telling him he was running late and anytime now the spotty lad with glasses is going to ask a question just to make things worse..., and then it was gone.

David Gray the spirit walked slowly back to where Alf sat. It had only been a peek, like dunking for an apple in a bucket of cold water, but the shock was the same.

'Anything interesting?' Alf said, eyebrows raised in expectation. Someone in the front of the audience asked a question.

'Disturbing, if anything, but no answers,' Gray muttered. 'It was dark, Alf, dark as night. I thought it'd be red like before, y'know, with the policeman and the major and that man in the park. I was ready to hear my thoughts and feel my feelings, but there was just blackness, a sort of black-blueness with points of light like..., yes that's it, like stars in the night sky.'

'Yeah?'

'Well that's what I saw, Alf. I couldn't exactly tell you what it means but I know that's what I saw. Take a look for yourself if you want.'

'You sure you don't mind?'

'Be my guest. I'd be glad of a second opinion.'

Alf was shyly hesitant. 'Can we do it together? It don't seem proper to look into yer 'ead without you being there.'

'I suppose so. It seemed roomy enough, and as far as I know, I've nothing to hide.'

Alf hoisted himself from the seat and the pair moved to the front of the room, positioning themselves on either side of Gray.

'Before we do this, Dave, take a good look at all these people listening and learnin' off you.'

He followed Alf's bidding, ranging his gaze over the upturned faces. Their eyes were all fixed on the man talking by his right shoulder; himself. At his body's right shoulder Alf stood with his long arm reaching out, pointing with a gnarled finger.

'They're why we're here, Dave. These youngsters are the future and you're shapin' it for them. Can't you see that? They're the ones who'll end up with Captain Whatsit on his starship. And they'll be doing it because you taught them.'

His jaw dropped. 'What! Just that. It's that simple?'

Between the two, Gray the man continued his lecture. 'What do yer mean, "Just that!". One of the most important things we do is teach each other, Dave. Otherwise there'd never be any progress would there? Remember that, it's important. Very important.'

'I suppose it is. I've always looked on it as just part of the job.'

'And so it bloody well should be. God, you can be a bit thick sometimes.'

'Sorry. I wasn't expecting something quite so simplistic.'

'Well it is. Now if you've finally got the message, Dave, shall we get on with looking inside yer 'ead. There's probably all sorts of crap and garbage in there that needs sortin' out.'

At the count of three they leaned in through his ears, left and right, and their faces met across an endless void filled with stars. Up, down and sideways, everywhere they looked was like a gin-clear night over a tropical sea, with countless billions of sparkling diamonds studding an ink-black canopy.

'Blimey,' Alf said.

Gray noticed no echo. Alf's voice sounded normal and his lips were moving, but he reasoned that since neither of them possessed a larynx, their communication was and always had been telepathic. 'Well, this is it, just as I said. But I don't think it's the real sky because I don't recognise any constellations.'

'Yeah, I see what you mean,' Alf said, gazing all around. 'It sure looks like *some* sort of sky, though, don't it?'

'Why isn't it all red, Alf? Like the others.'

'Dunno, mate. Perhaps it's because this is your 'ead and not someone else's. And it's where you said you wanted to look. It's in yer 'ead, not yer body.' Alf turned his face to the left, 'Look at that one, Dave, the really bright one over there.'

Gray looked, and the pin-point of light detonated into a moutain-sized disc - or perhaps his attention somehow magnified it - and on the huge expanse was an image of his youngest daughter as a child, playing with a hose on the garden lawn, innocently naked and squealing with delight when the water splashed her skin. It was a memory, a summer he'd almost forgotten.

'What about that one,' Alf directed him.

Whoomf; the first image collapsed as the next appeared. It was his wife Kate, young and beautiful in her nurse's uniform, walking down a corridor and gossiping with a bunch of other girls dressed the same. Gray felt a tightness in his chest. 'Oh, look at her, Alf. The one in the middle. Isn't she lovely? That was the first time I ever saw her; it must be almost forty years ago.'

Alf was enjoying the show. 'That one on the other side,' he said, indicating with a nod.

Gray found it, and immediately felt humiliated. It was another bright one, but the memory was of a frail old woman sitting at his desk in an out-patient

Chapter 7

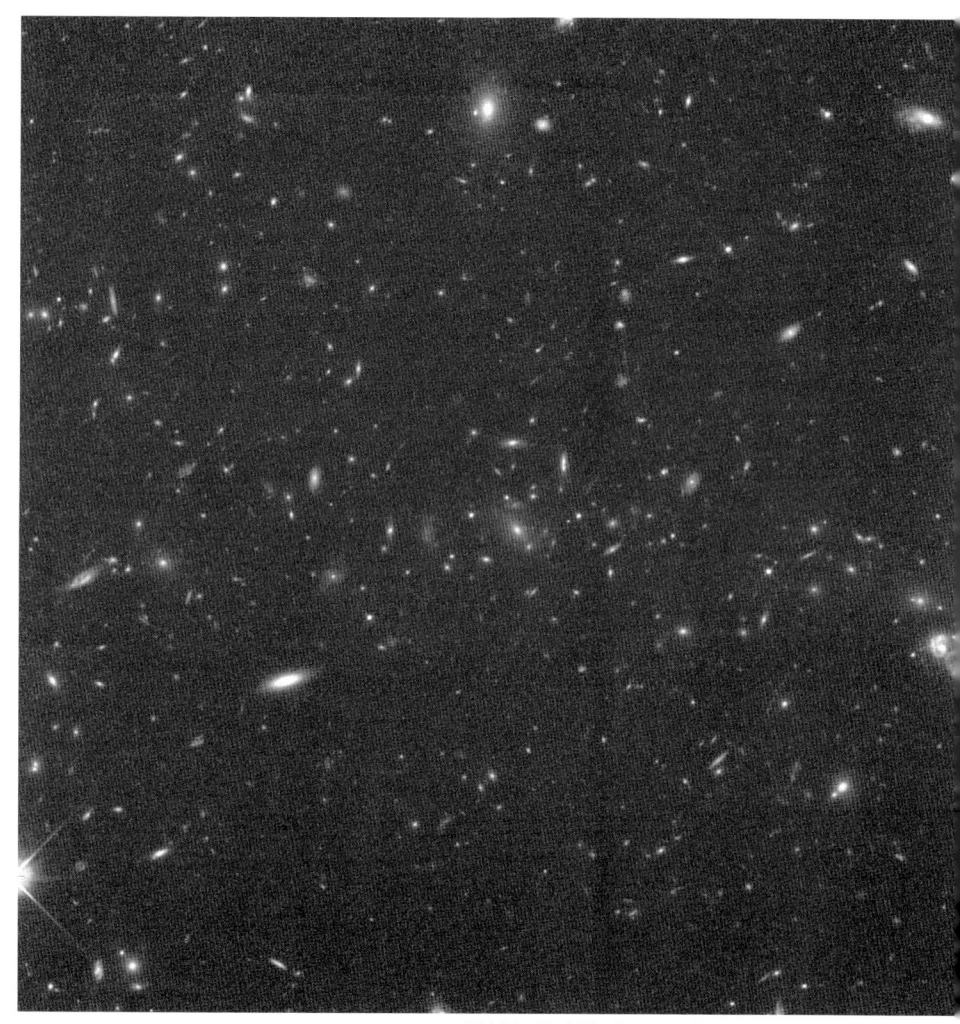

NASA: Hubble Space Telescope Center

clinic. He was a senior registrar - all crisp white coat with nothing more than a fountain pen - and on the wall behind him an x-ray film clipped to the fluorescent screen showed a colon cancer. His usual reaction would have been to relish the opportunity of adding to his growing total of bowel resections and book a date for her surgery, keenly looking forward to the technical challenge and the chance to polish his skills further. But that day, in that instant, he was overcome with sadness, both for the patient in front of him and the callous pride that had somehow inveigled his character. This unkempt widow who lived like a pauper without friends or family was more than just another left-hemicolectomy, and she didn't deserve another load of rotten luck. Her life was hard enough without having to undergo surgery solely for his amusement. He would have given anything to be able to wave a magic wand and cure her then and there, rather than be the instrument of further pain and misery. But he couldn't, and he felt wretched about it. So with a heavy compassionate heart he told an eighty-year old woman he'd do his best to cure her, because it was what she wanted to hear and because it was the only truth he knew.

Gray turned his gaze away and the image receded to a tiny dot among an endless vista of others once more. 'Alf, are these all my memories?'

'Reckon they must be, Dave. Amazing innit? All this space and stuff inside yer 'ead.'

In wide-eyed wonder Gray surveyed the infinite vastness of it all, though he purposefully avoided settling his concentration on any particular star - there were, after all, episodes in his life he would rather keep to himself. But with a bit of privacy, he reflected, it would be possible to spend a whole lifetime exploring this universe of memories. And as he looked, he remembered an average lifespan was something over two billion seconds - he'd done the maths as a schoolboy - and concluded these must be all his own. Then he peered downwards, and couldn't help being drawn to a particularly bright star, though it didn't explode into an image as the others had done. Instead, he felt himself falling. Falling towards it. And Alf followed alongside.

8

he front garden was much as they had last seen it, except it was now late morning and daylight. Having finished shoring up the house and brickwork, the workmen stood chatting in groups, smoking cigarettes, drinking mugs of tea and generally lounging around waiting for relief crews to arrive. The Jaguar, still embedded in the doorway but with its side guillotined open like a sardine can, held no occupant.

'Looks like they got you out, Dave,' Alf said.

'Yeah,' Gray murmured, his head finally clearing.

The trip from the infinite abyss back to the present had been a kaleidoscopic roller-coaster of sound and light. Mainly light, he recalled; the sound had been his own disorientated, involuntary screaming. But what a ride! Not through his memories though, as he expected, but through the very fabric of time and space itself. They had fallen through the universe, or at least, Gray's universe, and Alf seemed to have actually relished the experience, whooping with delight as they were hurled every which-way, tumbling through rainbow clouds of stars and convoluted bubbles of what looked like galaxies, swooping over elemental particles and vast whirlpools of glowing golden ether, tearing across fantastic peaks and troughs of undulating electric-blue waves. He had felt imbued with a wondrous joy and a privileged awareness of being a miniscule but fully integrated fraction of it. All matter, all life, all intelligence is ultimately derived from stardust and the Big Bang. Where had he read that? Understanding it from an intellectual scientific viewpoint was one thing. Appreciating it up close and physical, with a starting point inside his own mind was another.

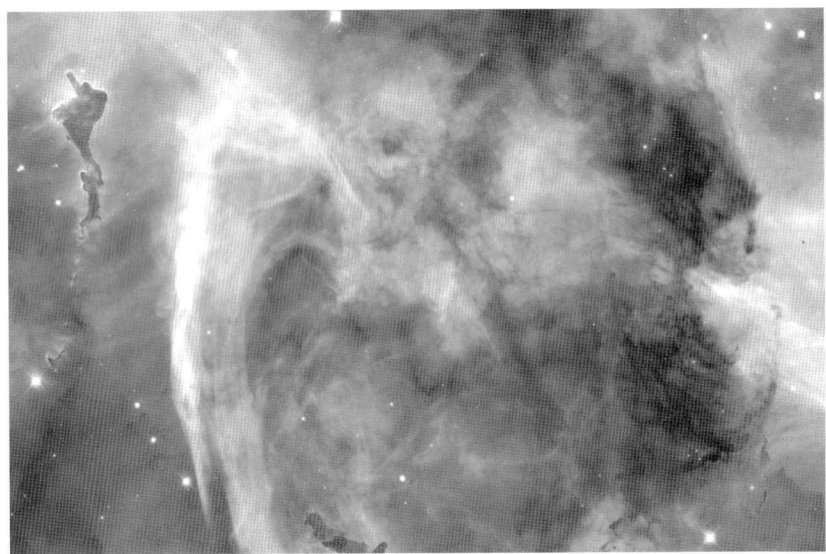

NASA: Hubble Space Telescope Center

It was part of him, and he was part of it; inviolably connected and whole, the self-same organism. Yet there was so much more to it than that. The root, the bark, the branch and the leaf of a simple tree can be recognised individually through the fingertips of a blindfolded man, but its magnificent completeness is lost to him unless he can step back and see it. And a tree without all of its parts ceases to exist. *Never send to know for whom the bell tolls; it tolls for thee.*

The disembodied consciousness of David Gray understood it all, recognised it intuitively. It was him, and he was it. And the knowing brought on an almost unbearable sadness for those unaware of the truth of universal being. How lonely, how isolated, how unfulfilled they must be in their blind ignorance. How infinitely magnanimous, how complete and wholesome, how eternal, how patient, is creation. Then the tears came. And he wept gently for the man he had once been.

'Come on, Dave,' Alf said, gently placing a comforting arm around Gray's shoulders. 'We made it back okay, didn't we? Don't get so upset.'

'I'm not upset.' Gray looked to the floor and rubbed his eyes, embarrassed.

'I know you're not, me old mate,' Alf said with a far-away smile. 'It was beautiful wasn't it? I wouldn't have missed that for the world.'

Gray giggled and pinched the bridge of his nose. 'That's such an understatement, Alf, you've no idea!'

Alf squeezed Gray's shoulders before letting go with a huge guffaw, 'Yeah, you're right.' He was pensive for a moment and then quietly exhaled, 'I just ain't got the words for it, Dave.'

'Neither have I, Alf, neither have I.'

Each smiled stupidly at the other in silence. They were brothers of sorts, fashioned from the same stardust to learn the same lessons, and experience the same emotions. It had been that way since the beginning. It would be that way forever.

Around them the workmen changed shifts, exchanged information regarding demolition and salvage plans, packed and unpacked tools, checked drawings and mains-service diagrams, called depots on mobile phones, gave out orders, worried about pay-cheques, and generally busied themselves with a thousand things of no consequence. And all the while, the Earth turned, and the sun climbed higher in a blue, blue sky.

'What now?' Gray said eventually. 'I'm clean out of ideas.'

Alf shrugged. 'Strangely enough, I could murder a cup of tea.'

'I don't think I can stretch to that, Alf. Space-time travel and enlightenment, yes. Tea no.'

'You'd better call up ma, then. She'll know.'

'Me!' The expectation of what the Katharine Hepburn duplicate might have up the sleeve of her prim cotton blouse induced in Gray a feeling of mild panic. 'Isn't that your job?'

'Not on your nelly, mate. This is your show, remember?'

The discussion might have continued for some time but was both unnecessary and futile, since the mere mention of Alf's mother delivered her into Gray's mind with the sharpness and surety of a six inch nail through the temple.

At once she was standing between them, eyelids narrowed, and with the hint of a smile on her thin, stern lips. 'Ah! So here you are at last. I thought we'd lost you both for good. Whatever possessed you?'

'Sorry, ma,' Alf sounded apologetic, but simultaneously gave Gray a confused enquiring glance.

The matriarch caught the gesture and deigned to expand further. 'We call it the universal memory loop, Mr Gray, a dangerous place which can suck you in forever. A few souls try it, but they're mainly foolhardy youngsters like you, who live with regrets and think they can go back to correct what they perceive as misdemeanours instead of simple lessons. Once caught up in the loop of one's own memories, a soul can be trapped for all eternity.'

'Oh.' Gray swallowed hard, recalling the temptation to explore memory after memory had been almost overwhelming. 'It was my doing, Mrs Angel, please don't blame Alf.'

She fixed him with a sublime far-away gaze. 'I know it was, Mr Gray, and I'm not blaming anyone. You were driven by curiosity to try to look into the future. It was expected you would, and that indeed is what you experienced. The youth who asked the question at your tutorial. Do you remember him?'

'Vaguely, Mrs Angel. The one with the glasses?'

'Yes. Eventually you will be his muse, and he will become a Nobel prize winner for services to medicine. But it was clear the memory loop was always going to be a grave hazard to you, hence the provision of a wise old soul as your temporary guide.' She nodded deferentially towards her son.

Alf? Mad Alf, wise? Speechless, Gray shot stunned looks between the two before concentrating on his unlikely friend. Alf's face bore a bemused smile, and despite the pyjamas, the wrinkles, the grey whiskers, the thinning unruly hair, his features *did* exude wisdom. It was there in the portals to his soul: powerful, fathomless, intensely cobalt-blue eyes.

Chapter 8

'Alf?' Gray pleaded for some explanation.

'Don't look at me, Dave, I'm just a normal bloke.' He flicked his flattened hand a few inches above his scalp and whistled through his teeth - *over my head, mate.*

'But you enjoyed that ride through the universe, or should I say my universe? You weren't scared, Alf.'

'Dave, it's all our universe and all yours. Each of us sees and feels things differently don't we? So we all live in our own and each other's. There's as many universes as there are people, more probably. And why should I be scared, I'm already dead, mate, ain't I? Or at least I will be soon, so what can hurt me? In any case once we started, I did enjoy it, yeah. Where's the harm in that? Anyway, we had to get back here one way or another, and I reckon you got something out of it as well.'

'Enough!' Alf's mother coughed politely and turned her attention to Gray. For the first time he noticed her eyes had the same forceful quality as her son's. 'You have many questions, Mr Gray, but since they are your questions, only your own answers will satisfy, so you must find them within yourself. I believe that process has already begun.'

With a lingering, knowing look, she then turned to her son. 'You have done well, Alfred, but your task here is now finished. Mr Gray will not require a guide for the remainder of his excursion and you have business of your own which you must attend to. A body cannot release its life-force unless the spirit is present to accept it, at which point one becomes whole again. So you must leave us now because your time is near.'

Alf opened his mouth to protest, but the sudden surprise on his face brought his lips back together. He felt himself being dragged away by an unyielding force, sliding backwards down a helter-skelter into a tunnel of darkness, with the bright disc of reality contracting in the distance until it was gone.

Gray looked on in astonishment as the solid form of his friend became translucent and was gone. Then he rounded angrily on the matriarch, 'We didn't even get a chance to say goodbye!'

'Why should you need to?' she asked coolly, one eyebrow raised.

'Because I might never see him again!' he yelled, and felt like adding "you silly cow," but thought better of it. Besides, he was concerned the workmen surrounding them might overhear his heated words.

She regarded him with the benign air of an eternally patient teacher. 'Will the sun rise tomorrow, Mr Gray?'

From his vantage of total incomprehension, he could answer no better than, 'As far as I know, it will.'

She smiled kindly and whispered, 'Correct.' Then she too became a wisp of light and vanished.

oooooooooooooooooooooooooooooooo

Gray studied the garden. It had been a typical suburban expression of affluence; a neatly trimmed lawn surrounded by flowerbeds of fashionably colourful shrubs and perennials, each geometrically orientated in a stilted regimented manner which ordinarily would have offended his aesthetic wayward nature. Now it was a mess of mud and bricks ploughed-up by heavy machinery, tyre treads, hosepipes and boots. A prick of guilt touched him. Not for the damage caused, but for the hurt and inconvenience the owners would go through when they returned from holiday and had to deal with it. And yet, what did it really matter in the enormous scheme of things?

One of the workmen was sitting alone on an intact portion of the low garden wall, intermittently drawing on a cigarette and surveying the scene from beneath his hard hat. Gray walked over to stand next to him, and took a deep breath.

'You can't hear me, can you?' he shouted

There was no response, other than the workman idly adjusting his balls through the crotch of his greasy jeans.

Gray sighed and let out a humourless chuckle. 'What a pity. All the things you could know if only you had the ears to listen.' He cupped his hand and this time yelled into the man's ear, 'I surfed through the universe and it was wonderful!'

The man hawked, spat out a gobbet of phlegm and took another drag on his fag.

'You're too engrossed in this illusion aren't you?' Gray stuck his chin up at the world in general. 'Too busy with material things, wasting your life away scraping a living in order to keep body and soul together.' He laughed with a bitter sadness at the unintentional truism buried within the cliché, and was immediately overwhelmed with pity. 'I'm sorry,' he said, pinching his eyes closed against tears. 'You're no different to anyone else I suppose. Too busy to smell the roses or look up at the stars.'

The workman stubbed out his cigarette under a heavy boot, stood up, stretched, farted, and then walked back to work.

Gray watched him go with a sympathetic smile. The one-sided conversation had left him feeling lonely, and he realised he missed Alf. And his wife, his darling Kate, what about her? Did she know he'd had an accident? By now she must do, he reasoned. What now then? Should he go home, or back to the hospital to check on Alf, his patient? Where would Kate be? He expected the unspoken questions to provide their own resolution with a whoosh to the chest, and blinked purposefully in the bright sunlight. But nothing happened; the view was unchanged. Trying a different tack, in his mind's eye he constructed the intensive care unit with Alf in one of the beds, envisaged the nurses milling around, heard the monitors' staccato bleeping, and imagined himself being there. Still nothing. For someone only recently introduced to thought transportation, he was both surprised and irritated he couldn't make it work, and reckoned the absence of his spiritual companion was somehow responsible. So, with mounting disquiet and a sense of forlorn abandonment, he shoved his hands into the pockets of his jeans and began walking.

It was ten miles or thereabouts. Out of the suburbs, into the city, back to the hospital, and straight to Alf's bedside. He had to get there, had to find Alf; wise old Alf would have the answers. To what? No matter. Just walk.

He flirted with the idea of hopping on a bus, or hitching an anonymous lift by stepping into a car halted at red lights. But how could any vehicle transport his insubstantial form? If he did get into a car, as it moved off wouldn't it simply leave him behind, passing through his body just as easily as he had passed through the metalwork in the first place? Holding onto something wouldn't help either - after all, he couldn't even sit on a park bench without sinking through it. There was nothing else for it, he would have to leg it all the way.

Moving unseen by pedestrians on the sidewalk, Gray effortlessly quickened his pace. Freed from the constraints of a hungry metabolism demanding oxygen and carbohydrates, he discovered he could not only walk, but jog, or run, or sprint, tirelessly. Not bad for a fifty-eight year old, he congratulated himself. But it didn't last long. On the city outskirts the roads and pavements were swarming with people, and he found it impossible to avoid them. The repeated shock of inadvertently blundering into one body while trying to avoid another - briefly having his vision blurred red and simultaneously sensing their sometimes horrific thoughts - slowed his progress to an ever wary, ever dodging crawl.

To escape the ordeal he took to the less crowded sidestreets and zig-zagged across town, steering clear of any further collisions by anticipating the glassy-eyed intentions of passers-by, predicting their movements, and side-stepping them. It was a solitary miserable chore, and he began to long for a simple nod of acknowledgment from a fellow human being, yearned to see a glint of recognition in a friendly face, a fleeting smile of companionship. But they all ignored him. He was invisible and therefore didn't exist.

By late afternoon it was dark, and with the absence of any warmth from the January sun, a misty dankness pervaded the air. Gray's route took him by the city football stadium, a huge construction of blue-painted steel and brick, nestled incongruously within a maze of narrow streets and terraced houses. Standing by the main gate, indistinctly picked out by the lights beneath the huge "Home of the Blues" sign, was a small solitary figure. Gray realised with a start it was the first person he had seen for... how long? He couldn't remember. Half an hour perhaps? Consumed by his own despondency and the need to find Alf, he had lost track of time. Not that time had any substance to it, he reflected, nor it seemed, any particularly regular track. He crossed the deserted road to the far sidewalk in order to give the lone soccer fan a wide berth; it would be safer than risking bumping through another body. Not far to go now, a few miles at most.

'Hello,' the stranger called out. A female voice.

Gray didn't bother even to look up, the greeting couldn't possibly be for him. Hundreds, if not thousands of people had ignored his presence all day. Why should this one be different? Without breaking step he walked on.

'Hello,' louder this time, and more insistent, 'Doctor Gray.'

He stopped dead. Well no, perhaps not dead. Dead would be a rather gauche term to use in the circumstances wouldn't it? Let's just say that with no mass and therefore no inertia, he stopped abruptly, turned slowly and then peered across the road at the interloper. The lights above the tall wrought-iron gates of the stadium entrance illuminated her from behind, turning her silhouette into a black depthless shadow. But around the slim dark figure he noticed the lazy mist dancing sinuously, like an incandescent silver halo.

'Yes?' he whispered.

'I've been waiting for you.' There was a hint of humour in the gentle statement.

'You can see me?'

The head appeared to nod. 'Of course I can. It's been a long time.'

Curiosity drew him nearer, but as he approached, she withdrew further backwards into the blinding light until he could barely make out her shape.

'Who are you?' Gray spoke as if to a frightened animal, soft subdued tones of safety and security. If she was to be his only contact with anything approaching humanity, he didn't want her scared and running away.

'Come closer,' she said, receding into the darkness beyond.

Turning his head slightly to shield his eyes from the glare, he stepped forward into the pool of brightness.

'Good,' she said from the inky shadows beyond.

Gray thought he recognised the voice, but couldn't place it. 'What do you want? Do you need help?'

The laugh was high and girlish. 'Always the gentleman. No thank you, David, I don't need help. It's more the other way around. Look behind you.'

He glanced over his shoulder and saw the entrance gates; he was now inside the stadium, having passed through the ironwork while concentrating on the girl and blinded by the light.

'Please forgive my trickery,' she said, 'but I wasn't sure you would consciously walk through them, and I needed to persuade you to follow me.'

'Why?'

'For a surprise.'

'What surprise?'

In an exquisitely embroidered golden sari, with yellow trinkets glinting at her ears, neck and wrists, she stepped out of the shadows into the light; a young and beautiful Indian princess. The effect seemed miraculous. Clasping the palms of her hands together as if in prayer, and smiling with unabashed delight, she slowly bowed to him.

'Chitra?' he gasped.

'You asked me not to leave you, David, that is why I am here.'

'Uh?'

She flashed an impish grin. 'In the hospital before I died. Don't you remember?'

He shook his head, dumbfounded.

'One day, you will. Anyway, I didn't leave you. I've been with you ever since. Always.'

'Always?' He felt his cheeks flush.

She bowed her head again, this time seriously. 'Privacy is respected.'

'But why, Chitra? Surely you've better things to do?'

With crossed arms she walked in a slow pensive circle around him, weighing her words carefully. 'Because you cried for me, and tears are very important. Because everyone deserves a guardian spirit. Because you're a good kind person. And,' she giggled, 'it was a choice between you and a boring old greengrocer whose only interest in life was short-changing his customers. So I chose you.'

He stared at her incredulously, his lips moving like a fish out of water. Eventually he managed, 'Everybo... But... How...?'

She tapped her temple with a slender forefinger. 'That voice in your head isn't always your own you know. Those cartoons with a little red devil on one shoulder and a heavenly cherub on the other aren't far wrong.'

'But that's impossible. I've never heard you!'

'Quite!' She raised her perfect eyebrows. 'You can be a very stubborn and difficult person. What we call insensitive, not tuned-in properly if you like. But if I shouted loudly enough, well...' She shrugged her shoulders.

'When?'

'Countless times. Which jobs to take, what house, which girlfriend, who to marry, but mostly, David, mostly, when to bite your tongue and when to apologise for being blunt and rude.'

Gray dropped his head repentantly, immediately recognising his own shortcomings. 'Oh dear. I'm sorry to have put you to so much trouble.'

'No matter, it's been fun, and the most important thing is that you've learned humility. So everything's going to plan.'

'There's a plan to all this?'

'Of course. You don't think the universe is a dumb accident, do you?'

Gray observed his inquisitor closely. A fifteen year old girl with an intimate knowledge of his life, his private thoughts, his failings. Yet her dark brown eyes held the same radiant quality he recognised in Alf's, so in spite of Chitra's apparently young age, no doubt she was another "old soul". How then to answer her question? Was it a test of some sort, or a simple statement? How to describe the nagging itch in his psyche which had been there since he was old enough to reason? The irritation which quietened if he ignored it and got on with life, but became infuriatingly uncentred when he tried to locate and scratch it.

He wrestled with it again now, in the glow of her benign and patient gaze. The elusive emptiness in his heart which made him feel less than whole. In truth, his lifelong interest in science was driven by it, but threw up more questions than answers. Newton's clockwork world didn't exist - never had done - though as a schoolboy he embraced the comfortable concept as a drowning man clings to a piece of driftwood. Then he learned, amongst other things, that if the charge on an electron differed by just a miniscule amount, nobody would be around to measure it. The so-called anthropic principle: things are as they are simply because if they were any different we wouldn't be here to pose the question. What a meaningless copout! Like hushing an inquisitive child with a "Because it is!"

So he turned to medicine because there he found some solid ground; tangible organs with recognisable diseases and proven treatments. And then to surgery, because like carpentry, it was honest manual toil which seemed to satisfy a nameless need. But then the itch returned. Only this time it was more fundamental than pondering the nature of elemental particles.

What is life?

How can breathing sentient creatures be alive one moment, yet dead and decaying the next? The collection of cells we call a human being will survive on a heart-lung machine, but the body itself might still be "dead", its essence gone for whatever reason gets written on the death certificate. Even individual cells, given the correct nutriment, live and reproduce indefinitely. Biologists have used eponymous "HeLa" cells as guinea pigs for decades, but they were originally harvested from a woman called Helen Lane who "died" of cancer. So where is her essence now: scattered piecemeal around the globe in countless laboratories, intact and elsewhere, or non-existent? And what about those people - usually the elderly - who announce simply that they've "had enough", turn their face to the wall and seemingly decide to "give up the ghost?"

Life he reasoned, must be more than biological, and "cause of death" just as big a copout as anthropism. The spark then, the essence, is surely Descarte's *cogito ergo sum:* consciousness and the ability to think and reason. But if that were the complete answer, we would all be clones of each other, yet we are clearly not. Even natural clones - identical twins - are discrete beings with their own thoughts and values. In other words, each has a different conscience.

So, he eventually concluded, life is consciousness coupled with a conscience of varied sensitivity; the variation explaining individual perception and choice between what might be described as good or bad.

'You've known that for years, David,' Chitra gently chided him from a distance of two yards, though her mouth formed no words. She was inside his head. The sensation was familiar and comfortable.

'Yes, but now I've seen the proof for myself, haven't I? But there's more, isn't there? Since my trip with Alf I feel lighter and bigger somehow, puffed upwards and outwards until I can hardly feel the edges of my own space.' He formed the words in his mind. 'It's as if all my senses reach out further.'

'Perhaps your consciousness will eventually stretch across all time and all space.'

'Even if it did, Chitra, I think I'd still feel there was a hole in my heart. It's like having an itch I can't find and can't scratch.'

'Don't you recognise what it is?'

'Well, I've never been entirely sure. And I know this sounds stupid because I love my wife and family dearly, and they love me. But it feels like...'

'Longing for an unrequited love?' She finished the thought for him.

'Yes! Stupid, isn't it?'

'No, because that's what it is. Disconnection from your first love. Your original mother.'

'The universe? All creation?'

'Every single thing. That's why humans search for true love from each other. But it's only a fraction of the real thing. The more you learn and understand, the more connected you become and the less it hurts. The plan is the driving force.'

'The plan?'

'Yes.'

'Should you be telling me all this, Chitra?'

'You were getting there by yourself anyway, and I think your own guardian is entitled to give you a little push. In any case, you can't learn from being told can you? What is it you tell your juniors when they ask for help? I believe it goes something like: "Get on with it your bloody self or you'll never learn".' She felt his embarrassment and laughed out loud. 'And then, then you stand outside the operating theatre doors spying on them and fretting like an old mother hen to make sure they're okay. You're just a big old softie.'

He felt the light brush of her lips against his cheek, though she was still standing out of arm's reach. 'Thank you, Chitra, I don't deserve it.'

She dismissed his comment with another beaming smile. 'Now for your surprise. And another lesson.'

'But I thought seeing you was my surprise!'

'No, but it's nice of you to say so.'

Gray expected to be whooshed away somewhere, but Chitra simply turned and led him across the broad expanse of tarmac towards the turnstiles. After a reassuring glance, he followed her through the locked doors and unlit corridors until they walked out onto the turf and stood alone in the centre circle of the playing field. The unique and seldom afforded viewpoint had him curiously studying the shadowed empty ranks of terraced seats, and for a moment his imagination took him off into every manchild's fantasy; playing professional football in front of a home crowd of screaming fans, beating five defenders to score the winning goal, and being feted as man of the match.

She saw the child-like wonder on his face. 'Penny for them?'

'Uh? Oh sorry, Chitra, I was just... Hold on a minute!' He gave her a sly look. 'You know already, don't you?'

Her eyes sparkled with amusement. 'Brilliant goal by the way, I didn't know you were so good.'

Chapter 8

'Yeah, it was, wasn't it?' he agreed. 'But what an experience it must be, Chitra, on the field with all those people cheering from the stands!'

Immediately it was bright daylight with fifty-thousand or more cramming the terraces. In the middle of the otherwise empty field, Gray stood alongside Chitra, transfixed by the scene and the wall of sound assailing his ears. Slowly he turned on the spot, taking it all in, comfortable with the certainty that both he and his companion were safely invisible. Impressive though it all was, why was this his surprise? It certainly looked like a football crowd, but on closer inspection he noticed there were no partisan colours, no flags or banners, no painted faces and hats.

'What's happening, Chitra, where are the teams?' Gray shouted above the din.

'There aren't any,' she spoke in his head again, her voice calm and reassuring.

'No football match?' his mind answered her.

'No.'

'Well, why are all these people here?' He waved an arm towards the sidelines, and at once the crowd went wild, redoubling the already deafening noise. With a start he realised they could not only see him, but were responding to his actions. 'Chitra?' he flashed the unspoken question once more.

'For you of course.' Her voice was tinged with a palpable mixture of joy and pride, and whether it was purposeful or accidental, she transmitted her emotions along with her thoughts. Gray found the sensation intoxicatingly blissful. 'Most are spirits like me, some are asleep and dreaming this episode, and others have the ability to transport their consciousness. But they are all here because you have touched their lives. This stadium is merely a convenient demonstration. No man-made structure could ever be large enough.'

'Chitra, that's impossible. I couldn't know even a fraction of them.' He scanned the incomprehensible numbers.

'Nonetheless,' she continued. 'They're here for you. Think about it! How many people do our actions affect in a lifetime? Every smile, every frown or

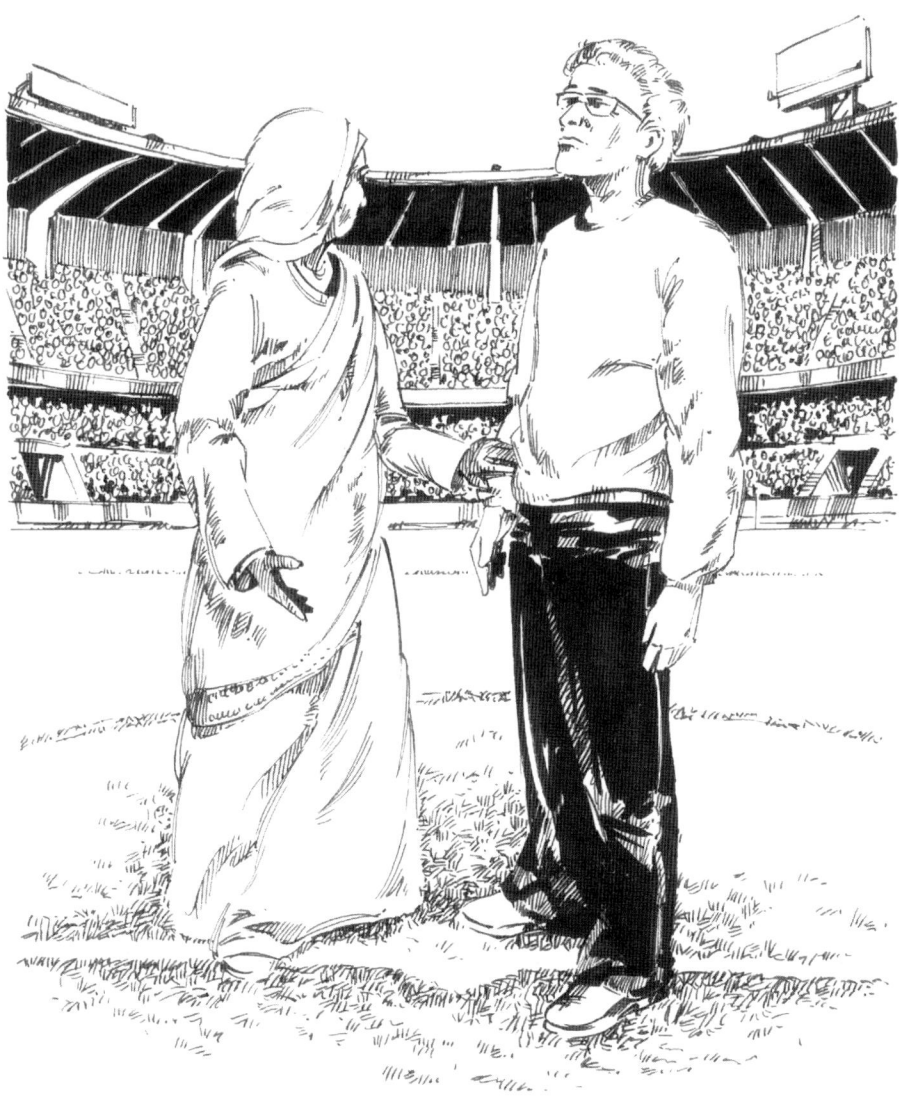

harsh word, every thought or intention, every deed good or bad, is a pebble thrown into an endless ocean. The splash is most noticeable to those nearby, but the ripples go on forever, influencing others in ways we never even consider. Doesn't that remind you of anything?'

He thought for a moment. 'Chaos theory? The flap of a butterfly's wing in Brazil causing storms in Japan.'

'Got it in one!' she nodded. 'But it's not chaos is it! Once we grasp that everything, every single thing, is connected, order appears out of apparent chaos. Every action has a reaction, every effect a cause. Now take something obvious like your job as a doctor.'

'Oh please, Chitra, don't start telling me I save lives, you of all people should know that's nonsense.'

She held up a slender finger to halt his objection. 'David, would you agree that at least some of your patients have lived longer than they would have done because of you?'

Gray was so caught up in the moment he failed to notice the crowd's noise hush to a dull murmur. 'Yes,' he conceded. 'But any half-decent surgeon would produce the same results as me, that's the nature of the job isn't it? Relieve pain and suffering and with the right disease you get living longer as a side effect. Bowel cancer is a perfect example. It can kill you from a blocked gut there and then, but remove the tumour, relieve the blockage, and in most cases you live long enough for it to kill you by spreading elsewhere, usually the liver, and that's a horrible way to go! It's not just cancer either. A ruptured spleen from trauma, a clot on the brain, even transplant surgery. Whatever. Get the message? The real question is, are we doing them any favours? What right does anyone have to make people live longer just so they can go on to suffer further pain and ignominy, which we all do, and inevitably end up dead anyway?'

She flinched at the statement, but said nothing.

Gray caught her expression, 'Okay, okay, Chitra, not dead, go through the "transition".'

'How many of your patients have ever objected to living longer, David? How many have begged you not to treat them?'

'Very clever, Chitra, but tell me this,' he countered. 'How many truly realise they never really die? How many, if it were possible, would look into the future and see it's going to be so painful they'd rather not to go there? And how many, knowing all that, would there and then opt out and ask for the morphine and scotch treatment to help their "transit"?'

She smiled serenely at his outburst and slowly inclined her head, but again remained silent.

'Exactly! It's as if we've all been brainwashed to cling onto our body at all costs. Why? Life is consciousness and conscience. If only everyone appreciated it, flesh and blood would lose its importance. And for that matter, so would wars, murder, greed, deceit, materialism, and all the other dreadful things mankind's capab.... '

A sharp prod in the back brought his mounting tirade to a sudden end, and Chitra brought a hand up to her mouth to hide a fit of giggles. Gray spun around to spy his assailant, 'What the ...?'

In a sports jacket and flannel tousers, with a silk cravat tied carefully above the open neck of his checkered shirt, the man looked every inch the elderly country squire, including the meticulously Brylcreemed short hair and burgundy face.

'Look here old chap, if you don't mind me saying so, although some of what you say is correct, much of it is complete tosh,' he said, waving a deer-horn walking stick at Gray like a sword, though a moment earlier it had been used as a cattle prod. 'Think straight man, work it out properly. If you're nothing but consciousness and conscience, and I'm not disagreeing with you there, why bother to be born? Eh? What's the purpose of it? That's the conundrum you should be working on.'

Gray blinked with bewilderment. 'Er, excuse me, have we met?'

'Yes, but I doubt you'll remember. You operated on me thirty years ago for a burst ulcer or somesuch. Happily I survived that skirmish and eventually died from a heart attack at my proper time. I for one would like to thank you

Chapter 8

for giving me those extra years, both the good and the bad. And so would they.' He pointed his stick towards the crowded stands and was rewarded with a thunderous ovation.

Gray looked upon the massed throng, and shook his head. 'All these people can't possibly be patients of mine!'

'No, no, no. Of course not. They're with me.'

'What, all of them! Who are they?'

'A few of the people affected by you saving my life. Thirty years is a long time.'

'You must have been pretty famous then,' Gray said without thinking.

'Not at all,' he guffawed. 'Just a normal chap thankfully, though I have to say that early brush with death, the one when you saved me, did alter my perspective on life somewhat.'

Chitra's words glided back into his mind; "Ripples in an endless ocean", and at once he understood some of it. She was standing next to him now, thanking the man for his co-operation, thanking him for gathering together his extended family and friends and acquaintances, and their families, and their friends and their aquaintances, and so on...

And then it was dark once more, with Gray and Chitra alone on the football field surrounded by deserted terraces.

'That was a good question he asked,' she said.

Gray was still looking around, stunned at the sudden transformation. 'Eh?'

'Why bother to be born?' she repeated.

The soft beguiling voice grabbed his attention, and he looked down to concentrate on her innocent almond-shaped face. She had died so young, before her life even got started, missing out on love, and motherhood, and a thousand wonderful things. A hint of the original sadness from all those years ago shivered through him, and with a stunning insight, he understood that by witnessing her brave fight for life, and subsequently her death, she had left her mark on him forever. And knowingly or unknowingly, each day since, he had passed it on to others, in his words, in his deeds, in every handshake and smile, in every "How are you?"

'Why indeed?' he whispered. 'Why did you, Chitra? Why did you bother to come into this world for such a short painful time?'

'We each have our own reason, David.' She smiled with perfect pearl-white teeth, teasing him. 'But mine is no longer important. Tell me, why were *you* born?'

'I don't know, Chitra. I've never thought about it that way. The meaning of life, yes, I've pondered endlessly over that one. But turning the question on its head like that, and asking why was I born?'

As the words left his mouth, the ground beneath his feet vanished as surely as if he'd stepped off a cliff, and Chitra's upturned smiling face shrank to a distant speck until it was gone. Like a dimly remembered childhood nightmare, he fell backwards, enveloped in an endless tunnel, down and away from her, accelerating wildly, arms and legs flailing, clenched teeth suppressing the screams in his throat until he could no longer hold them, and they escaped unbidden, long and loud and howling.

And then, with a gut-wrenching thud, all was stillness and quiet.

And pain.

9

Gray hurt. Everywhere. Legs, arms, belly, chest, and a sledge hammer was doing its own thing inside his skull. Something was in his mouth, slithering down his throat like a serpent, hissing rhythmically into his lungs, and with each expansion any number of broken ribs creaked agonizingly. Carefully, slowly, he tried lifting his eyelids, and was rewarded with a monocular view of a white ceiling with fluorescent light strips and more pain; his left eye stayed swollen shut. So he closed his good eye, retreating once more into darkness, and concentrated on his hearing. No pain there at least, and the sounds were unmistakably familiar; bleeping monitors, the regular shush of ventilators, hurried footsteps, doctors giving orders, nurses shouting instructions, the hum of air conditioning, thumping noises.

Beneath the fingertips of his right hand he recognised a cotton sheet, and the thing invading his mouth - he stroked it with the tip of his tongue - was an endotracheal tube. He was in an intensive care unit. No doubt about it. How did he get here? Think!

But his brain wouldn't work. The pain was intolerable, the noise distracting, and both competed for his undivided attention. So he concentrated on the inside of his eyelids and withdrew from his senses, gently dropping beneath the clamorous assault on his ears, and then deeper still, below the level of his pain, until he found a deep comfortable place to be alone.

He found Alf there, waiting for him, still in his pyjamas. "Ello, Dave. You made it back then!'

Gray found he was carrying a bedsheet, and wrapped it around his naked body like a toga. 'Looks like it,' he said with a genuine smile of recognition. 'God knows how though! Nice to see you, Alf. Didn't think I'd get another chance.'

'I'll always be here for you, Dave, whenever you want.'

Gray looked around. They appeared to be in white space; no form, no depth, just a gentle ambient illumination. 'Where are we anyway? Where exactly is here?'

'In yer 'ead mate, I thought you knew. Mind you, yer imagination's got a lot to be desired ain't it?' Alf cast a critical eye about the place. 'Is this all you could dream up?'

'What do you fancy?' Gray said, catching the mood and the implied request on Alf's roguish face.

'Surprise me.'

And then they were in a meadow on top of a hill overlooking rolling countryside, the hot summer day alive with the trilling of larks and the hum of myriad insects. In the hazy distance a glittering river meandered towards the coast on the horizon, and fair-weather cumulus scattered the sky.

'Nice,' Alf said. 'Very nice.'

'Holidays in Southern France,' Gray explained, sitting on the ground to admire the view.

Alf followed suit, and the scent of wild flowers and crushed grass lifted to his nostrils. 'Wow!' he said, inhaling the sweet air approvingly and leaning back on one elbow. 'Smells as well! You're good, Dave!'

'My pleasure.' Gray smiled, and for a while the pair sat in companionable silence, each knowing this was goodbye. High above, Gray added a dozen wheeling swallows to the scene and studied their aerobatics. 'What happens now, Alf?' he said eventually, afraid of spoiling the moment.

The old man sighed, and his rheumy eyes glistened brightly. 'Well, right now, upstairs, or downstairs, or outside, or whichever way you like to imagine it, in the bed next to you, they're jumping up and down on the empty body I used to live in. There's a terrible fuss going on, electric shocks, injections, the whole works. Is it always like that?'

'Yes, it's organised chaos.' Gray laughed out loud at the deeper truth in his spontaneous reply.

'Wasted effort though, ain't it? 'Cos I'm here and whole again.' Alf grinned, but his expression was tinged with sadness.

'You're leaving, aren't you?'

'It's time, Dave, I can feel me ma pullin' at me. Don't know where she is, but she's out there somewhere and I reckon she's found me another job to do.'

Both men rose slowly to their feet and bearhugged each other. Gray felt a pleasant tingling sensation before he stood back, aware that even in bright sunlight, Alf's glow was more pronounced than ever.

'Au revoir, Alf, and thanks.'

'It was fun, Dave, so it's me who should be thanking you.'

The pair shook hands and then Alf hitched up his pants, turned his back, and started walking downhill, whistling happily to himself as his bare feet negotiated the gentle incline towards the valley below. Gray watched him go with bittersweet emotions churning in his chest, and waited for his new-found friend to turn and wave a final goodbye.

But if he did, Gray didn't see it. After a hundred yards or so, Alf's luminescent outline, diminished as it was by distance, crossed the dazzling light reflected from the surface of the distant river, and the two seemed to merge until Gray was forced to look away from the glare. And when he looked back, Alf was gone.

For a fleeting moment Gray remembered a question he'd wanted to ask, but then the noise and the pain took hold again.

ooooooooooooooooooooooooooooooo

Admitting the on-call senior surgeon to his own hospital following a road traffic accident caused quite a stir and raised a number of problems. In line with usual practice, the paramedic crew phoned the casualty department to warn they were bringing in a major trauma case, thereby allowing twenty minutes to bleep and assemble the trauma team; namely the surgical, orthopaedic and anaesthetic registrars, their respective juniors, the x-ray staff, and any other available casualty doctors and senior nurses. As soon as the trolley was rushed into the "majors" room, the well-practised crew descended like hungry vultures onto the unidentifiable blood-soaked occupant, and then recoiled in electrified horror when, after cutting away the filthy clothes and temporary bandages, the shattered body of Mr David Gray was uncovered.

This revelation struck the surgical registrar particularly hard, but it wasn't because a few short hours earlier he'd been assisting this human being to do a leaking aneurysm, though that was shocking enough. Nor was it because he found himself in the unenviable position of having to treat a more senior colleague. His main concern, above all others, was that the mangled unconscious mess in front of him was also his boss; the man he was supposed to call for help, if and when he landed himself in the brown stuff. Judging by the extent of the injuries and the rapidly distending abdomen, this was such a time. In more ways than one.

First, he brought a halt to the temporary inactivity. 'Come on, get on with it people, let's have business as usual. Follow the trauma life support protocol, head to foot films, cross-match, neck lines, all of it. You know what to do.' Then he spoke to the night operator on the hospital switchboard. 'I don't care how you do it, but get hold of any consultant general surgeon other than Mr Gray.'

Pause. 'But Mr Gray is the surgeon on duty, doctor.'

'Yes I know that, but he's…, unavailable. I need one of the others. And while you're at it, you may as well wake up whichever anaesthetist and orthopod is on tonight.'

In the event, once the surgical registrar explained his dilemma, most of the consultant body arrived to help: anaesthetists, surgeons, orthopods, physicians, neurosurgeons, ICU specialists; the lot.

David Gray spent four hours under the knife having bones in his legs pinned, a dislocated hip reduced, a ruptured gut repaired, a collapsed lung inflated, one arm plastered, and numerous lacerations sutured. CAT scans of his head and brain showed minor contusions but nothing needing the skull cracked open, so the disappointed neurosurgeons were sent home. The chest injury and fractured ribs necessitated six days on a ventilator with appropriate sedation, analgesia, intravenous feeding and antibiotics.

One morning, a week after the initial injury, the ICU staff decided the contused lung was sufficiently recovered to discontinue sedation, stop the ventilation and remove the endotracheal tube. With his vocal cords free to vibrate, Gray could at last speak rather than mime, though every breath felt like fire.

'My wife,' he wheezed.

'She'll be in to visit later, Mr Gray. She know's you're going to be okay. Now lie back and rest.' The nurse spoke in a patronising childish voice, and he concluded she couldn't have been more than twelve years old.

Because of his status within the hospital, Gray was afforded a plush room and concentrated medical care from his consultant colleagues, physiotherapists (whom he renamed physical terrorists), nurses, occupational therapists, nutritionists, social workers, and all manner of allied services. Including his wife.

'I want to come home, Kate.'

'Oh David,' she cried, resting her head gently against his chest to hide the tears. Gray stroked her hair with his one good arm. 'I want you back so much, but you're not ready yet. I know it's horrible in here, but please stick with it a little longer, darling. I thought I'd lost you once already. I haven't the courage to risk that again.'

He was in hospital just over four weeks in all, slowly graduating from bed to chair, to wheelchair, to crutches. From tube feeding to fluids, from being spoon fed, to feeding himself. From catheter and bedpan to a commode, and then finally, gloriously, to a proper toilet. But while he struggled with his healing body, an even bigger battle raged in his head.

Did it actually happen, or was it all a dream; the product of a rattled and bruised brain? And how to tell Kate? Would it comfort her to know death was just a transition and she could never lose him, or would it frighten her into thinking her husband had gone barking mad from a knock to the head? Indeed, should he dare to tell anyone at all, and if he did, would it result in psychiatrists being added to the constant stream of visitors?

The pre- and post-traumatic amnesia wiped clean almost two weeks of memory. He had no recollection of the accident or the days before and following, yet strangely, the adventure with mad Alf and all the others was as real to him as the broken nose on his face, and discrete enquiries confirmed he had indeed done an aneurysm on a man called Alfred Angel.

'It was weird, boss,' his registrar explained during a detour from his ward rounds. 'He was in one bed, you were in the next, and there was I looking after both of you. Pity he died really, it would have been hilarious to see the patient visiting his surgeon instead of the other way around. Y'know, I really thought he'd make it too. No bleeding, kidneys okay, and then he ups and has an infarct on us. We crashed him but he never got going.'

'Any family?'

'Seems not. I passed him over to the coroner but he was happy not to have a post-mortem. I think the Borough Council dealt with things after that.'

After due deliberation, seasoned with sizeable chunks of self-doubt, Gray finally decided to keep quiet about his near death experience. From what he had heard and read, it was in any case unlike any other, and everyone knows a concussed brain can play strange tricks.

When they eventually allowed him home, his wife treated him like some rare Fabérgé egg; a particularly delicate one with a cracked shell. She insisted on "feeding him up" with nourishing broths, limited his ration of malt whisky and cigars, "I'll allow you to smoke in the house for now", cut short visits from his children and grandchildren before they "tired him out", and generally fussed in an overly loving way. Initially, he revelled in all Kate's attention and thrived, but after a month, as his strength returned, he felt trapped and bored to distraction. Except at night. That's when the dreams came.

Crazy, ludicrous dreams of picnics alongside his favourite gin-clear trout stream, with cold meats and strawberries and pastries and chilled white wine, all spread out on a chequered cloth laid on the ground beneath glorious blue skies, and so real he could taste the food and dabble his bare feet in the cool water. Of themselves, such dreams in a man starved for so long of fresh air and simple pleasures are hardly worth mentioning, and indeed, one might say are probably to be expected. But what made Gray's phantasms so noteworthy were the guests.

Each successive night, three or four of them - but never more than there were place-settings for - would stroll along the river bank, thank him kindly for his hospitality and settle in a circle to enjoy the meal. With mounting amazement Gray discovered he was entertaining all manner of dead medics from the renowned to the unrecognised, yet the agreeable and light-hearted banter covered ordinary everyday topics like medicine, politics and the parlous state of the world and the health service. Indeed, the same sort of prosaic chat heard whenever and wherever doctors congregate socially.

'And what do you think, David? Are you an advocate of this new-fangled laparoscopic surgery?' Alexander Fleming helped himself to a large slice of ham and smeared it with mustard.

'I think it's great for gall bladders and hernias,' Gray said. 'Other than that,' he shrugged, 'I suppose I'm a little too old to see the logic of spending half a day doing an operation which ordinarily takes me an hour or less.'

'But isn't the plan eventually to get robots to do it?' The lady was called Liz, and she had spent her life as a paediatrician before being knocked off her bike and killed by a drunk-driver.

'I think that's years away yet. The big thing at the moment is distance operating. With a video link it's possible to sit in London and do an operation in New York using computer-assisted robotic instruments, but there's always a trained surgeon pulling the strings.'

'Yes, I've seen that. It's quite remarkable,' said the public health doctor from China whose name Gray couldn't get his tongue around.

He tried quizzing them about their experience of life and death, the nature of consciousness, good versus evil, and other metaphysical issues he wanted resolved, but they all either politely ignored him and changed the subject, or gave him a look which said he should know better than to ask. Eventually, with the wine and food gone and the sun dipping down to the horizon, his guests would say their goodbyes and wander off into the distance, calling out promises to all meet up and do it again one day when Gray became a dead medic and joined the Society. But as he watched them go, though inspired and excited by the characters and their intellect, a nagging doubt always plagued him, and each morning he woke restless and unfulfilled: surely these people have better things to do in heaven?

The final dream - about the twentieth, though he didn't then know it would be the last - had only two place settings laid on the chequered cloth, and instead of Gray's normal casual clothes, he was wearing his fishing kit and carrying his favourite rod and reel. It seemed the most obvious and normal thing to do; tie on a likely dry-fly from the wallet in his pocket and pass the time away until his guest - whoever it might be - appeared. Shielding his body behind the lush mid-summer reeds and bullrushes, Gray crept down across the meadow to the wide gently flowing stream, all the while studying its glassy surface for the tell-tale ripple of a rising trout. He'd done it since boyhood, and always, always, he took the whisper of his grandfather's voice with him.

There! Near the far bank, ten yards upstream. Wait lad, be still, be patient. Yes, there it is again. Spluch; what a gloriously soft sucking sound they make as they take the fly. Okay, carefully get some line out with a few false casts downstream where he can't see it dazzle in the sun, then punch it forward and land it light as a feather six foot in front of his nose. Don't aim at the water, aim above it or you'll splash. Oh my Lord, thank you, thank you, it's perfect. Absolutely perfect. Now mend the line, boy, pull in the slack as the fly drifts down, keep in touch with it but don't let it drag or the ripples'll spook the fish. Here it comes now, floating over the spot, the exact same spot. Yes, couldn't be better. Steady now, steady, wait for it. Spluch!

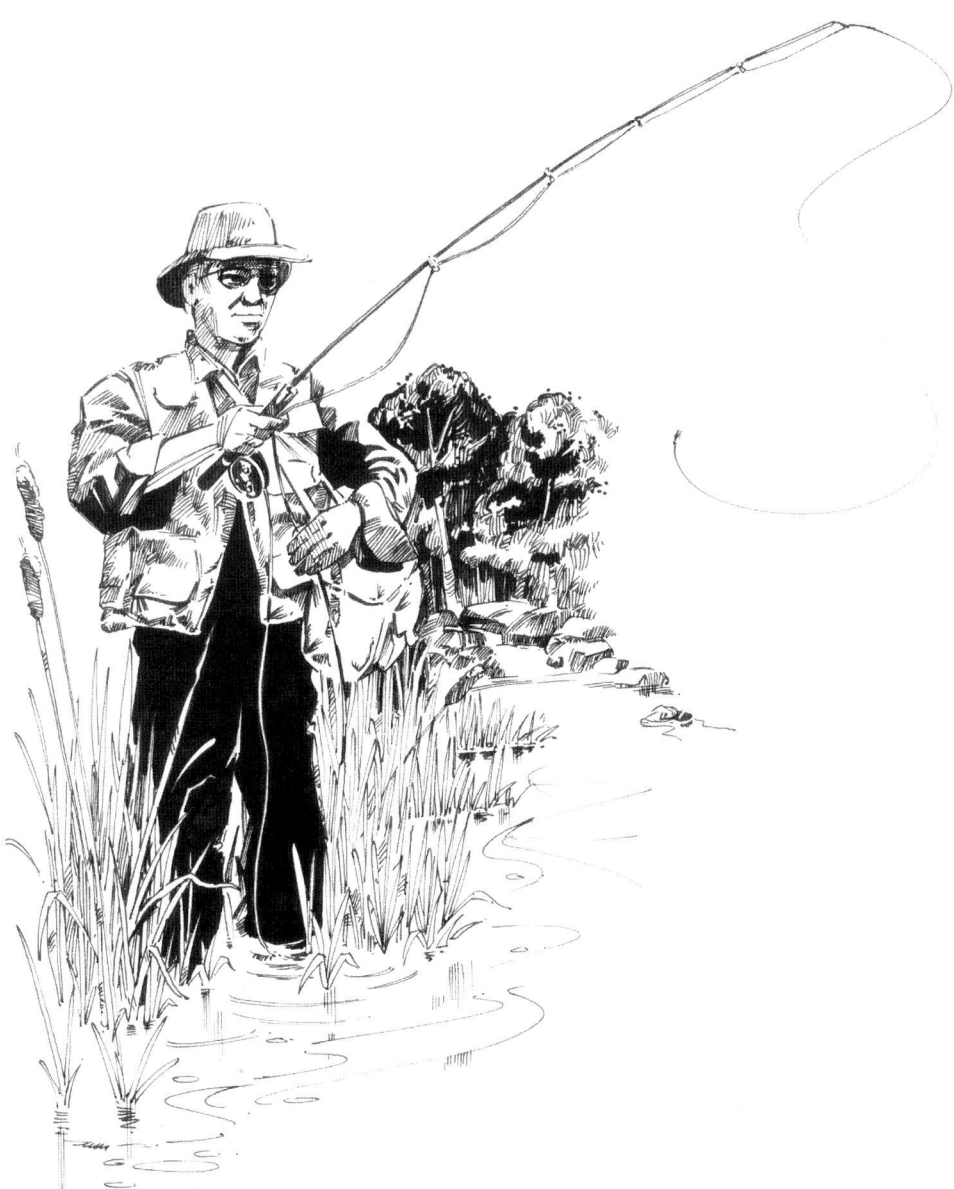

Five minutes later Gray was gently cradling the foot-long wild brown trout within the cup of his hands at the surface of the water's edge. As ever, he thought it breathtakingly beautiful - an irridescent slab of polished bronze glittering in the sunlight, fading at the belly to a deep butter-yellow, with the flanks tantalizingly bespeckled in jewel-like spots of ruby, amethyst and pearl. 'What a lovely creature you are. Two, no, easily two and a half pounds. You're not the biggest brownie I've ever caught, but thank you all the same for making my day. Now off you go home, and be more careful in future.' Gray opened his fingers, the trout flicked its large tale, and was gone. Attempting to follow its passage through the water he knew was a futile task - the outrageously colourful camouflage was faultless - yet with his wet hands shading his eyes, he tried all the same.

'You still can't bring yourself to kill 'em, can you, lad? And tell me, what are you going to say when one eventually talks back to you?'

It had been forty years or more, yet he'd half-anticipated, half-hoped this was the reason; why else would he find himself fishing? Gray turned his head slowly for fear of losing the moment.

'No need to worry, lad.' The Yorkshire lilt was just the same. 'I've been given a furlough for the day from your grandmother, and with fishing this good, I'm not going anywhere soon.'

Gray splashed from the stream to where his grandfather stood on the bank, all business-like in thigh waders, and a waxed jacket and cap, with his ancient Hardy split-cane rod grasped in one hand and a dead trout dangling by the gills on the index finger of the other. It was an image he'd always retained, an unspoiled timeless register somewhere in his memory, in that universe of stars. He threw his arms around the shoulders of the short round figure, and hugged him until they were both breathless. Gray had watched this same man melt away from cancer of the prostate, and then his grandmother, whom he loved with an equal passion, died six months later from heartbreak, though the certificate had said pneumonia.

Chapter 9

'Grandad! I knew it'd be you. I just knew it. How are you both?' Gray stood back at arm's length, embarrassed by the uncontrolled and spontaneous physical expression of his love, but his hands held on tight to his grandfather's shoulders. It had been so long since they'd touched, he wasn't yet prepared to let go.

'We're both fine, lad, so there's no need to fret yourself. More to the point, how are you getting on, and where's the lunch I was promised?'

Gray led the way towards a nearby oak tree under which lay the picnic cloth with its array of delights. Before sitting down his grandfather plucked a few large dock leaves from beneath the closest hedgerow, and tenderly wrapped his trout in them before gently placing the green package in the deep poacher's pocket of his jacket. 'Your grandmother told me she wants at least one for the pot,' he explained, shrugging off the coat and hanging it in the shade on one of the tree's branches.

'You're as bad as you ever were,' Gray said, teasing him. 'You hate killing them as much as me.'

'That is true, David, my lad, but at least I don't talk to them. And when you've known a woman as long as I have, you'll understand the true meaning of bribery and corruption.' He winked mischievously. 'Now then, let's eat, I'm famished.'

Gray was delighted to be sharing some time with his grandfather, and even though it was a dream, his beaming grin was uncontainable. The man in front of him, gnawing on a chicken leg and recounting tales of long-distant fishing days, had once been a rural general practitioner, happy to take payment in cash or kind, or often accept nothing at all. He was also the larger-than-life character who mentored and encouraged Gray to go into medicine in the first place.

'Anyway, enough about fishing,' his grandfather said, suddenly serious. 'I understand they've been at you to join the Dead Medics' Society.'

It was an unexpected question, and Gray stumbled with the answer. 'Yes. How on earth did you know that?'

'Your name came up at one of our meetings.' He put the now bare chicken bone down and picked up a glass of Chablis. 'I wouldn't want to influence you unduly, lad, but I think when your time comes it would do you good to become a member, at least until Kate joins you. They've an excellent social and support programme, and if you fancy dabbling in research or acting as a muse, there's an active scientific group too. They're sure to find a man of your experience something useful to do.'

Gray ruminated on his grandfather's words, and his eyes filled with quiet tears of intense sorrow. 'You're telling me I'm going to die before her, aren't you? And I always hoped to go second, to save her the pain of loneliness.'

His grandfather took a sip of wine, seemingly unconcerned. 'Within the context of infinity, David, I promise you it's not a great problem, so don't get upset. Maybe Kate needs to learn that pain, if only for a short time. Suffering is good for the soul you know, including the onlookers. And unfortunately, you will have to watch her suffer, as I did with your grandmother.'

The kindly fisherman kept his gaze fixed intently on his grandson's tear-smeared face, and chose his words carefully. It was an onerous task the DMS had thrust onto him, but he was the only one courageous enough and close enough to be able to do it. 'Tell me, do you want to die now, lad?' he said gently.

'No!' Gray yelled.

'So why do you want to live?'

'To be with Kate, of course.'

'Why?'

'To spend time with her, to love her, to learn from her, to enjoy our life together.'

'And what do you think your patients want?'

The exquisitely distilled simplicity of the statement had Gray sobbing uncontrollably into his fists for a while. It was all so obvious, so clean and uncluttered. When he eventually looked up his grandfather was still there, watching over him with a gentle smile. 'Thank you, grandad,' he whispered.

Chapter 9

'It's my pleasure, lad. Oh, and by the way, in spite of what I've just said, you won't be parted from Kate for a long time yet, you've both still got some learning to do. And don't forget, young Toby is going to need someone to show him how to fish, isn't he? Though it's a pity his grandfather is a bit of a second-rater compared to your own.' He smirked in anticipation. 'Do me a favour though, David. Please don't teach the boy to talk to them, it's so humiliating.'

Gray laughed out loud, the previous sadness overwhelmed in a floodwave of affection.

'Now before you go, there's someone I'd like you to meet. The instigator of your enlightenment, so to speak.' He put two fingers to his lips and whistled loudly. Across the meadow, at the base of the far hedge, a fox pricked up its ears and began trotting easily and purposefully towards them, its reddy-brown coat and white bib contrasting sharply against the emerald pasture. At the edge of the picnic area it sat on its rear next to Gray's grandfather and looked into the man's face with all the devotion of a labrador, tongue lolling from its mouth and panting in the heat. He stroked its head. 'This handsome fellow is the fox you killed. He's become rather attached to me, but I can't think why.' He winked slyly at Gray, reached towards a plate, and handed the animal a drumstick. The fox took the juicy tit-bit in its mouth and made off in the direction it came from. They both watched it go.

'I knew a fox was involved, but I can't really remember the accident,' Gray said. 'Glad to see it's safe and well though.'

'Guessed you would be. He keeps me company whenever I come fishing, though between you and me, I think it's only cupboard love.' He laughed. 'Haven't thought of a name for him yet, but he answers to "boy" well enough, so I probably won't bothe...'

Gray awoke in his bed and reached out in the darkness to cuddle the sleeping form of his precious soulmate, Kate. However long they had left together, he determined at that moment to relish and enjoy every minute. By the time the first rays of daylight crept through the window, his dream was no more than a fond and distant memory.

OOOOOOOOOOOOOOOOOOOOOOOOOOOOOOOOOOO

At the first promise of spring, with daffodil shoots studding the broad lawn and primroses brightening the flower borders, Gray sat at the window of his study and came at last to a firm decision. He had to find Alfred Angel. 'Lord knows why,' he sighed to himself, and lifted the phone.

The coroner's officer at the hospital explained the legal niceties and confirmed his hopes. Burial rather than cremation with the costs coming out of the estate of the deceased: 'Just in case someone shouts foul, Mr Gray, then the body can still be exhumed for forensics. With no beneficiaries, the taxman takes whatever's left over.'

Once through to the mortuary, the senior technician congratulated his old friend for sounding so well, asked when he was returning to work, and expressed regret that the fridge he had reserved was never used: 'Yes, you know, the big one at the end of the row, only the best for you, David. But never mind, perhaps another time, eh?' Then, with howls of laughter echoing over the line, he checked the logbook and furnished the name of the undertakers and the date the body was collected. One more call and the hunt was almost finished. Gray knew which cemetery to visit.

But it was more difficult than anticipated. Kate refused to allow him out of the house alone, and insisted on taking him. 'Why are you doing this, David?' she said with a sideways look from the driving seat.

Why indeed, and how to explain the disquiet in his heart to this loving, darling woman? Though she denied it, the last few months had pushed her to the limit; he saw it now in the lines on her brow and around those pretty green eyes. Should he add to her burden with the truth, or fudge it? Being anything less than candid felt wrong - thirty-five years together was a long time - but in all honesty, he couldn't discern fact from fantasy.

'It's difficult to say, Kate. I'm not hiding anything because I don't understand it myself, but something's bugging me. The fact is, I've got a two-week hole in my life and I think this man Angel has something to do with it.'

'But how?' she pleaded, anxiety rising in her voice. 'He died on the night of your accident didn't he?'

Chapter 9

It pained him to see her worried face; he had already said too much. 'No, he survived almost two days.'

'So what?'

He shrugged his shoulders. 'Let's just wait and see.'

It was threatening rain when Kate parked and helped her husband from the passenger seat to his feet. Under a low forbidding April sky, favouring his good leg and supporting the bad one with a crutch, Gray shuffled along the neat gravel path towards the rows of newer graves. At his insistence Kate sheltered in the car, watching his slow painful progress through moistened eyes.

He wanted, needed, to do it alone. It was a matter of honour. A solitary pilgrimage to the grave of a man who had become his friend; a man he never knew in life, apart from to plunge a knife into his belly.

And then he found it. A cheap and simple stone with no motif. No cross, no wings, no flowers, no epitaph; just the name, age and year of death.

'Not much is it? The Council didn't exactly splash out, did they?' he muttered into the wind self-consciously. 'Never mind, Alf, I'll get you a decent one.'

'Forget it, Dave, it don't matter, I ain't got any bleedin' attachment to it have I?' The voice inside his head was familiar and welcome, but the shock nearly knocked him off his feet.

'Alf, Alf is that you?'

'Who else were you expectin'? It's my grave, ain't it?'

'It was all real then. I didn't imagine it?'

'What do you think? Isn't that why you came here?'

'Sort of. And to pay my respects.'

'There's no need to go to all this trouble, mate, you can talk to me whenever you want. I told you, I'll always be there for you, just call. How's the pain by the way? You've been through a rough time.'

'I'm getting there.'

'Good. Now, what is it you really want, Dave? I can sense you're troubled.'

'It's something Chitra said to me. Oh sorry, Alf, do you remember Chitra? You saw her soon after we...'

'Yes, Dave, I remember Chitra, and I've met her since. We had a long chat before she handed you over. Smart girl that one.'

'Pardon? What was that about handing over?'

'Ma decided I should look after you from now on and give Chitra a rest. I said it'd be a pleasure, which it is. Good the way it works, innit?'

Gray considered the prospect momentarily; a close friend available in his head to talk to and discuss things whenever he wished, one who's judgement he could rely on, and one, unbelievably, he could actually hear! It felt good somehow, sort of cosy and safe. But there was another implication, one with a little sadness attached to it. 'What about Chitra then, is she redundant now?'

'No way. She's been given a youngster who needs her, a little boy in a family with more trouble and strife than you could shake a stick at. You were getting too old and wrinkly for her anyway. What you need is a grisly old bastard like me.'

Gray followed Alf's humorous lead. 'Well, ancient master, I'm very honoured, but I have a question for you.'

'Shoot.'

'Why was I born, Alf? I don't know and I can't work it out.'

Hysterical laughter echoed somewhere between his ears. *'Yer daft bugger, no-one can tell you that can they? You have to find it inside yerself. That's like askin' someone why they climbed a mountain. Sometimes even after they've done it they still can't or won't say. And 'appen they'll go back and do it again and again in different ways, or climb another one, for the view, the challenge, the crack, the rush, the achievement, or simply because it's there. Who knows? All of it and more probably, but at the very least they can say they've done it, enjoyed it and learned something, even if it's how to cope with being scared.'*

'Is that it? All of it?'

'Well, there is one more thing. When you've realised why you were born, you'll know, and you won't want to climb mountains no more.'

'Well, what about you, Alf. Do you know why you were you born?'
No answer.
'Alf...?'

'David darling, are you okay?' Kate's concerned voice whispered from behind and to one side of him. Her approach had been unseen and unheard, and Gray realised with a start that his eyes were closed shut, the better to concentrate on Alf's ethereal advice. He opened them now and spun around to look at her. The fear and concern in her face cramped his heart.

'Better than ever, kiddo!' With a broad reassuring smile, he gathered her in his arms, kissed away her tears, and then crushed her gently into his chest until the moment passed.

When Kate eventually stepped back, she rested her hands on his cheeks and examined her husband's bright eyes at arm's length. This man was the love of her life; she knew every line on his face, every nuance of his handsome features, and could read him as easily as you read this now. 'You are better aren't you?'

Gray nodded. 'I've just got a load off my mind.'

'Because you found him?' Cocking her head to one side she examined the gravestone at his back, 'Alfred Angel?'

He grinned. 'I'll tell you all about him when we get home.'

She briefly looked again, and shook her head in amused disbelief. 'Unusual inscription isn't it?'

'Eh?'

'Haven't you seen it?'

'Of course I have, it's nothing special.'

'Then I think you'd better look again.'

On the headstone, below Alf's name, where before had been flat featureless stone, was written:

A Wise Old Soul

ooooooooooooooooooooooooooooooooo

It took Gray a further two months to claw his way back to something resembling good health; good health that is, for a man approaching sixty. Even then, his leg ached if he'd been on it continuously for more than a few hours, and he took to using a walking stick on ward rounds and favouring his one good leg when operating. But he never once complained. Instead, he regarded the disability as a constant reminder of his adventure with Alf, and the extraordinary revelation which had been gifted to him. He would never die. No-one ever died.

This absolute certainty imbued his life with a supreme and joyful composure which infected all around him. Everywhere he looked he saw people with their own mountain to climb, for their own reasons, using their own route, and most importantly, needing enough time to do it. This insight gave him the wisdom and caring to lend a hand wherever and however he could, to ease their path and help them on their way. And he came to think of himself and his fellow medics as purveyors in quality life-*time*, considering the job well-done if his patients could face their final illness without mental or physical pain, and satisfied they had lived long enough to accomplish their desires.

And never again did he think a patient might be better off dead. After all, that would not only be disingenuous, but impossible.

Gray tried to explain his epiphany to his wife and a few close friends. They gasped in wonderment at his tale, but the condescending lob-sided smiles always betrayed their scepticism, even as inside his head, Alf's voice echoed: *"Don't fret, Dave. They'll know when they know. Just give 'em time."*

As any mortal might, he contemplated retiring. After all, he had good enough medical reasons to, and the pension would have been more than adequate. But for the new enlightened Gray, time became a precious commodity, not something to be squandered on the vegetable patch or world cruises. He was here to learn, as he always had been, and, as ever, his patients were the best teachers. Gray came to understand compassion as just one glittering facet of an even greater gem; a gem with caring, truth, charity, kindness, friendship, devotion, and a thousand other expressions of mankind's benevolence etched indelibly onto its surface. A huge gemstone called love.

'Are you sure it wasn't all a dream, darling?' Kate said alongside him in bed one evening.

'Even if it was, it doesn't alter the lesson does it? Think about it. All the religious claptrap in the world surrounds one central theme, one simple truth: death isn't the end, and every holy man, every guru, every sage and saint in history have all preached the same. Life ever after is what we all aspire to, so why does everyone find it so difficult to believe? The rest is just philosophy or dogma clouding the issue.' He squeezed her hand to enforce the point.

'Here's a simple test,' he continued. 'Tell me, how old do you feel on the inside?'

'About twenty,' she said without hesitation.

He chuckled. 'Everyone always answers the same. I've even asked ninety-year olds and get the same answer. On the inside, everyone's twenty or thereabouts.'

'So?'

'We don't get old, Kate, even though for a short time we're trapped in a body that does. No-one feels any older than they did as a young adult, though I'm willing to bet there are a few people out there who'll tell you they're ancient, like Alf Angel, an old soul. We are infinite beings, Kate; we exist forever. Knowing and accepting that gives everything a different perspective. The pain, the heartache, the money worries, the pettiness we endure from day-to-day, all become as insignificant as a single grain of sand on an infinite beach of the stuff.'

'But David, each grain must have some importance, otherwise there'd be no beach.'

'Very good!' he purred in her ear affectionately. 'But every grain is a distraction to either get lost in, or learn from. In a million years from now, or fifty, or even ten, how significant will the mortgage be, or my car crash, or this present life? As long as we're together, strolling along that beach above it all, nothing else matters does it?' He kissed her cheek.

'What are we here for then?'

He kissed her on the lips. 'I can only answer that one for myself.'

'And?' She kissed him back.

'To learn how to love. Forever.'

My lamp is almost extinguished.
I hope it has burned for the benefit of others.

Sir Percivall Pott, 1714 - 1788

Author's note

Although this short tale is clearly fiction, the historical figures and operations depicted are real, though the characterisation is down to poetic licence. David Gray and Gerry Westman, rather than single individuals, are amalgams of many surgeons I've known - so don't bother to go looking, you won't find them. Likewise, Alf Angel isn't a real patient, he just arrived out of the blue one evening and began whispering into my ear as I sat at the keyboard. However, I must confess to a sneaking suspicion he really does exist, out there somewhere and willing to talk to whoever will listen. There's a line in a Nanci Griffith song which says it well: *Bring the prose to the wheel, I'm not driving these wheels today.*

During my research I came across many learned tomes, but the most valuable were those by Professor Harold Ellis; not only a famous surgeon and superb teacher of the craft, but also a prolific and lucid scribe with an infectious passion for his antecedents and their work. If you have a continued interest in the history of surgery, seek out his books.

And finally, if you haven't already spotted the inspiration, it's *A Christmas Carol* by Charles Dickens. He wrote his "ghostly little book" in 1843, and even if you know the story backwards, as we all do, I'm willing to bet you haven't read the original since you were at school. If the inclination takes you, do it again now or sometime in the near future, and then ask yourself this: how on earth did old Charlie, way back then, come up with the idea of space-time travel?

142 Dead Medics' Society